SEVEN
SECRET REASONS

WHY YOU CAN'T LOSE WEIGHT
AND KEEP IT OFF

ROB NELSON, MS

TAPROOTS PRESS

SANTA ROSA, CALIFORNIA

SEVEN SECRET REASONS
WHY YOU CAN'T LOSE WEIGHT
AND KEEP IT OFF

Cover image "Egg Rain of Spring" by Krista Lynn Brown © 2009
www.DevaLuna.com

Printed in the United States of America

First Printing, 2023

ISBN 978-1-7336826-2-6

Taproots Press
Santa Rosa, CA

www.TaprootsPress.com

Contents

Section 1: A New Understanding........................ix

1. Why This Book?......................................1

2. Core Concepts......................................9

3. Taking a Look Under the Hood 15

4. EFT Crash Course.............................25

5. Tapping for Younger Selves................35

6. Cultural Programming 39

7. Self-Loathing....................................45

Section 2: The Seven Secret Reasons 55

8. Binge Eating....................................57

9. Protection from Sexual Attention 67

10. Fear of Loss 77

11. Rebellion....................................87

12. Deprivation.................................97

13. Obsessive Thinking 109

14. Fear of Dating and Relationships............119

Section 3: Breakthrough Strategies 131

15. Cravings 133

16. Listening to Your Body's Wisdom...........143

17. Tapping Away Limiting Beliefs 149

18. Affirmations 159

19. Conclusion................................169

Appendix: Tapping Script from Hell 175

Resources 181

Acknowledgments..............................183

About the Author 185

Hacking Reality...............................187

*This book is dedicated to my beloved wife and soulmate
Krista Lynn Brown, my amazing daughters India & Eden,
and all the wonderful clients, students and colleagues
who've shared their weight-loss journey with
me, while attaining such profound
levels of healing.*

SEVEN
SECRET
REASONS

WHY YOU CAN'T LOSE WEIGHT
OR KEEP IT OFF

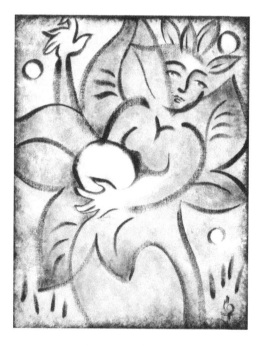

Egg Rain of Spring by Krista Lynn Brown

A New Understanding

Once the Secret Reasons are resolved, your set-point changes. Appetite and metabolism re-adjust to a healthy, ideal new setting. At that point, weight loss becomes automatic and inevitable. A non-issue. That may sound too good to be true, but I've seen this happen for clients again and again

Why This Book?

This book is different. You'll find nothing here about diet or exercise. No keto, paleo, low-carb diet recommendations. No supplements or superfoods or smoothies. No promises of magic bullets that miss the mark. If you find yourself frustrated, exhausted and deeply discouraged in your struggle with weight, this book may hold a surprising key.

This book is about discovering and eliminating the reason WHY you have a weight issue so that getting to your ideal weight becomes effortless and inevitable. Instead of endlessly trying to diet and exercise with discouraging results, you'll learn how to put your weight loss on autopilot. No more struggle.

I'm not talking about self-hypnosis or positive thinking. No. I'm going to teach you something new. Something that actually works – an extremely powerful tool called EFT tapping which focuses on resetting subconscious beliefs to effect positive change.

Tapping is an absolute game-changer and although it is scientifically grounded, the results seem almost magical. It's probably unlike anything you've ever experienced. EFT is also easy to learn and you can get to work right away, changing your subconscious settings for weight.

Why focus on the subconscious? Because it holds the missing key – the Secret Reasons you can't lose weight or keep it off.

The Secret Reasons

You want to lose weight, right? That's a *conscious* intention. Maybe you have an ideal weight or dress size in mind. Or you just want to drop 20 pounds. The reason it isn't happening is because your *sub*conscious mind has other ideas. It wants you to stay the weight you are, or maybe even add a bit. That's what you're up against.

This book explores the Secret Reasons your subconscious has to keep you overweight– and guides you through resolving them.

Over the years, I've discovered seven common Secret Reasons that keep my clients from losing weight. You might just have one, or maybe two of them. It's *very* unlikely you'd have all of seven! Unfortunately, one is all it takes.

Maybe it seems like your body (subconscious) hates you and wants you to suffer. I know it can really feel that way. But that's not what's going on! All of the Secret Reasons are misguided attempts to protect you, or heal you from old traumas.

In this book we're actually going to work *with* your subconscious, to free it from the past and actually change its mind. But first, let's look at *how* the subconscious is working against you right now.

Appetite & Metabolism

Your body has a "set-point" for how much you should weigh and I'm guessing that the setting is not to your liking.

What is a set-point? It's like the thermostat in your home or car. You set it for 68 degrees and it'll do its best to maintain that temperature, cranking up the furnace when it's cold out or switching on the A/C when it's hot and the sun is beating in.

Instead of a heater and A/C though, your weight is primarily controlled through appetite and metabolism. And despite your best efforts, your subconscious is the one setting the "thermostat."

Your subconscious controls your appetite – what you're hungry for and how much you want to eat. And it also controls your metabolism – how fast you'll burn the energy you take in, or whether you'll actually store that energy as fat.

You can *try* to take control of these factors consciously, speeding up your metabolism through exercise, and overriding your appetite with will-power and discipline. But let's face it, sooner or later you'll get tired and lapse. It's like trying to swim against an undertow. Or sometimes a rip tide! We get tired, but the subconscious never stops.

You were actually born with healthy settings for weight, along with settings for a gazillion other physiological processes in your body. It's *all* being run by your subconscious mind, and for the most part, that's great.

You don't have to worry about excreting just the right digestive enzymes, healing a cut on your finger, regulating your blood pressure, replacing worn out cells – it's all taken care of automatically.

But somewhere along the line, your original healthy settings for weight were changed. Readjusted. And not by chance. That's where the Secret Reasons come into the picture.

Because it's vastly more powerful than your conscious mind, this book is all about working with your subconscious mind, to change the thermostat back to the original healthy "factory default settings" you were born with. Once that's accomplished, weight loss will be automatic.

Until recently, *making* this kind of readjustment was pretty much impossible, but that's all changed with EFT tapping.

EFT - Emotional Freedom Techniques

EFT tapping is a way of communicating directly with the emotional part of your brain, where trauma lives. This is a really big deal, because that's a totally *non-verbal* part of the brain. You can't talk to it, because it doesn't understand spoken language.

That's why talk therapy is pretty much useless with any kind of trauma. Imagine a veteran with really bad PTSD, just back from Afghanistan. You could tell them "Hey, relax. You're home. It's okay, you're safe now." Would that be helpful?

Of course not! The part of their brain that holds the PTSD can't understand a word you're saying.

This is what makes EFT so different. We tap on eleven specific acupuncture points with our fingertips, while saying words that focus on what's wrong. This gets right into that non-verbal brain, discharging old stuck emotions and negative limiting beliefs. The first time I tapped, I experienced changes I didn't even know were possible!

You may have been carrying around guilt, anxiety, sadness or shame for years and years, and then with a little tapping, suddenly it's just gone. And *stays* gone. Old bad memories and traumas lose their charge.

This is how we're going to let go of any Secret Reasons that have been holding you back.

The tapping scripts in each chapter are designed to help resolve certain key traumas so that your appetite and metabolism can re-adjust back to their original healthy weight settings. At that point, weight loss becomes automatic and inevitable. A non-issue. That may sound too good to be true, but I've seen this happen for many clients.

Not only that, by going through this process of changing your subconscious set-point for weight, because it is all interconnected, you'll most likely upgrade *every* area of your life – relationships, work, prosperity, inner peace, creative self-expression. Everything.

What could be more helpful than resolving key traumas, releasing old stuck emotions, and letting go of old, negative patterns of thinking?

Our Adventure

This book is divided into three sections. We'll start out with the mechanics and dynamics of the subconscious mind and how you are being protected from your own desire to lose weight. There's also a crash course in EFT tapping that I hope will be life-changing for you.

In the second section we'll explore the Secret Reasons – where they come from, how they get installed and how to resolve them to get this junk out of your system. And even though not all of them will apply to you, this information might be helpful for friends and loved ones who are also struggling.

The third section gives you powerful ways to augment the freedom you're gaining, by tapping away cravings and letting go of limiting beliefs.

The icing on the cake, if you'll pardon the expression, is a chapter on affirmations and how to get them accepted by your subconscious using EFT tapping. If you've tried using affirmations in the past, to no avail, tapping is the game changer!

Because most of my clients over the years have been women, and especially those with weight issues, you may see that reflected in my stories and tapping scripts. That said, I do believe this book can be just as helpful for men.

This is NOT a diet book

I assume you already know what not to eat. But I'm *not* asking you to give up the foods you enjoy. It's time to start letting go of the struggle. No more titanic battles with cravings. No more being set up for failure because you're working against your Secret Reasons.

Instead, let me just ask you to pay attention to how you're feeling as we work our way through these chapters. Just a little homeopathic dose of mindfulness, perhaps. Along with that, I'd like you to practice regarding yourself with affection, and all of your "sins" with compassionate curiosity.

As far as what you *should* eat? I'm sure you've noticed there are a LOT of diets out there, many of them contradicting each other. Who knows what's right for you?

I believe that your *body* knows. Your body knows exactly the right food for you at any given moment, and as the background noise of negative beliefs, old stuck feelings, internalized media messages and trauma is tapped away, you'll be able to hear the quiet voice of your own body with increasing clarity.

And as your set-point readjusts toward an ideal healthy weight, your appetite will readjust with it.

You *Have* to Do the Tapping

If you want this book to work for you, you can't just read it. You're going to need to do the tapping. That said, some of the Secret Reasons may not apply to you, and you can just skip the tapping for them. But for those that *do* resonate, it's EFT that makes all the difference.

Tapping is wonderfully easy, but if you feel too intimidated, or you just can't bring yourself to tap, all is not lost! Check the resources section in the back to find qualified EFT practitioners who have trained with me and understand the Secret Reasons. Especially if you have devastating traumas to resolve, it's always best to work with someone good.

My goal with this book is to help you lose weight and keep it off effortlessly. But even more so, to live a happier, more successful and authentic life. Thank you for reading it!

CHAPTER 1

Core Concepts

Most people try to lose weight by managing their diet and sometimes exercising to burn more calories. I'll admit this can actually work sometimes, for some people. No question about it. Unfortunately, more often than not, their weight loss rarely lasts. Sooner or later the pounds come right back on.

One problem with this approach is the need for willpower and discipline. There's usually a struggle involved in resisting urges, cravings and temptations. Day after day, having to find the wherewithal to keep at it. As long as you're winning the battle, you get to feel good about yourself. One little slip-up though, and your self-esteem is in peril, and all your hard work may come undone.

Here's a question for you: if maintaining this kind of weight loss program is a struggle, who or what are you struggling against? Where are those cravings really coming from? Is there a discouraging voice inside that undermines your best efforts?

Losing the struggle might make you feel deeply flawed, unacceptably weak, simply not strong enough, a conviction that it's just your lot in life to be heavy. I'd like you to consider a different idea: that we all have different parts of ourselves and those parts may have conflicting goals.

The part of you that wants to lose weight and be healthy may simply be at odds with a much younger part of you who wants ice cream, and wants it right now! Is this who you're struggling with?

We're supposed to be the captain of our own ship, but sometimes there's a mutiny and things get out of hand. Remember Captain Bligh from Mutiny on the Bounty? He was such a severe disciplinarian, the whole crew turned against him. He lost control.

Do you tend to be harsh with yourself?

I don't know about you, but I've had the somewhat horrifying experience of seeing my own hand bringing a piece of cake toward my mouth, despite the fact that I'm already stuffed and don't really want it. Mutiny!

Who has access to my hand?

Younger Selves

There's a common pop-psychology notion of the "inner child." This may surprise you, but for our purposes I suggest you ditch that idea. It's just too vague and imprecise. Instead of an "inner child," what you actually have are Younger Selves. Plural. You have *lots* of them.

Your Younger Selves are parts of you that split off in some moment of great distress. They are trapped, endlessly reliving that bad experience, like a tape loop from hell.

For you that terrible moment is just a memory, but for that Younger Self it's a current event that never stops happening.

Each Younger Self is a part of you, but they don't really know *you* exist. They're not out to get you, but sometimes they do get their hands on the wheel, so to speak. Or on that piece of cake.

In fact, the more cut off we are from these Younger Selves, the more autonomous they become. And it's natural for us to want distance from any memory that holds a lot of fear, sadness and especially shame. But the more we push our Younger Selves away, the more independent they can become.

If current events (in our life now) happen to match the circumstances of a Younger Self's hellish experience, they are likely to be "triggered" and will often end up sabotaging us.

Ironically, we ourselves can trigger them. When you make a healthy decision to cut sugar out of your diet, for example, you're essentially stepping into a kind of parental role with yourself, right? Well, if you happened to grow up with a controlling or overbearing mom or dad, one or more of your Younger Selves may become activated, or triggered.

They somehow confuse you with Mom or Dad, and here comes the rebellion. Here comes that piece of cake toward my mouth!

Self-Protection

When our Younger Selves grab the wheel and we find ourselves eating junk, it usually feels like "self-sabotage." And it is! At least as far as losing weight goes. But that's another term I'd like you to toss out the window. It's way more helpful and accurate to replace "self-sabotage" with "self-protection."

Here are a few hypothetical examples of what I mean by that:

Amy is 47 years old and wants to lose 25 pounds. Her decision to go on a diet triggers her 13-year-old Younger Self, who experienced (and is STILL EXPERIENCING) some *very* unwanted sexual attention for the first time. In that moment of trauma, the 13-year-old actually decided to put on a lot of weight as quickly as possible, as a strategy to become *un*-attractive and therefore safe.

Even though this 13-year-old is unaware of her adult self, Amy's decision to lose weight (and thus become more attractive) registers as intensely threatening. The next thing you know Amy is binge eating!

Or take Mary, who grew up with an overbearing mom, who required Amy to look like a perfect little doll. Mary's decision to go on a diet registers with *her* Younger Self as potentially losing a bitter power struggle. Her thought "I'll be damned if I let mother win" now applies to adult Mary! Mary has become a stand-in for Mom.

Even if there's no real threat of unwanted sexual interest in Amy's life today and Mary's controlling mother died many years ago, their Younger Selves are each trapped in their own time. For them the threat never stops happening. Their need to feel safe or avoid having their will extinguished in a terrible power struggle, can easily trump our current needs and desires to lose weight – even if those current needs are real and pressing!

Our Younger Selves might actually "self-protect" us to death.

How to Proceed?

That's why our approach in this book will be to explore, discover and resolve any Secret Reasons you might have for keeping the weight on. We'll be exploring a number of them in the following chapters. Some may not apply to you at all, but one or more might.

Our Secret Reasons almost always come from Younger Selves trying to deal with an intolerable situation, so resolving this stuff usually means helping some of them with EFT tapping. This is not a job for Captain Bligh! To really help your Younger Selves it's best to meet them with the same kind of love and compassion you'd offer any child (or anyone, really) who's going through a crisis.

Weight loss becomes pretty much inevitable once your subconscious mind is good to go. Why? Because your conscious and unconscious goals are no longer in conflict. They're aligned and heading in the same direction. No more struggle.

In the next chapter we'll take a deeper dive into what's going on in your subconscious.

CHAPTER 2

Taking a Look Under the Hood

Th is chapter is a crash course on the hidden psychology that may be running much of your life. Especially whatever weight loss issues are getting in your way.

I'm sure you've heard the term "subconscious mind," but most people I meet really have no idea how powerful it is, or the incredible influence it has on how our life is going. Let's start with your physical body, where it's easy to see how the subconscious is running the show.

We're so used to our bodies, we may take them for granted. Honestly, the human body is probably one of the most complicated things in the entire universe. There are millions, perhaps billions of things happening in your body all the time, none of which require any attention from you. From regulating your blood pressure to secreting digestive enzymes, it's all running on autopilot.

Even if you wanted to influence one of these processes, like growing your hair faster, good luck with that! Maybe some yogi or monk, meditating for years high up in the Himalayas, has that level of control, but for most of us our autopilot takes care of business and that's a good thing.

If it ain't broke, why fix it? For the most part, having all of this stuff run automatically is fantastic. If we had to devote our attention to even a tiny part of digesting breakfast, replacing worn out cells in our eyes, healing a bruise or growing our toenails, it'd be pretty tough to get through the day!

All of these physiological processes are handled for us by the *sub*conscious mind. The prefix "sub" means under or beneath, like in "submarine," which means beneath the water. Sub-conscious means beneath the level of our conscious awareness. We're usually born with all the programs and settings for keeping our bodies running smoothly preinstalled. No need to learn any of it.

Learning the Ropes

Human behavior, on the other hand, *does* have to be learned. Only the teensiest fraction of what we do is instinctual. And we have to start learning it right away, as soon as we're born, while our brains are just getting started. This is a really big task. If you think about it, human interactions are enormously complex.

All of us have to *learn* how to fit into our own family, how to understand and speak their language. We have to figure out that a behavior that elicits love and support from Mom, may not go over well with Dad. Something that works in the morning totally flops at night. Being helpful makes Mom and Dad happy, but our sister gets mean.

Remember Tarzan? After mastering a very instinctual life, the Lord of the Jungle had to learn the rules of proper British society. These were very popular books, perhaps in part because they highlighted just how difficult it really is – learning how to fit in, having "manners" and behaving in a way that actually works with other people.

Learning to walk took some effort, but it was *vastly* simpler than figuring out how to get along, especially if your family was a bit dysfunctional. For some clients I've worked with, being raised by wolves might have been a serious upgrade.

At any rate, in those first 7 years of life, your pre-rational brain downloaded truly *staggering* amounts of information, mostly taken in through your eyes and your ears and all of it dumped into your subconscious mind.

Early childhood is a rather dreamlike, impressionable state, and we're unable to really question or challenge what's being taken in. With so much information to absorb and assimilate, we just don't have the luxury (or capacity) of picking and choosing what's valid, functional, or even true.

Clash of Two Worlds

Okay, so where am I going with this?

Your weight issue today represents a collision between your automatic, inherited physiology and some of that learned behavior you picked up as a child. The conflict between knowing when you're full versus a compulsion to clean your plate, between craving leafy green vegetables for strong bones versus chocolate ice cream after a stressful day at work.

Your body instinctively knows what *it* wants for optimal health and vitality, but other parts of you, also subconscious, may have very different agendas. That's what we'll be exploring in the next section of this book. So you likely have a clash between those two aspects of your subconscious, but also with your conscious intentions, your goals for a healthy and trim body. Kind of a three-way fight!

By the way, that conscious mind of yours is pretty awesome, right? That's the part of you that's awake and aware. The part that decided to read this book, thank you very much, and is even now taking in the information, seeing how it fits in with or contradicts what you already believe.

Our conscious mind enables us to entertain new and creative thoughts, and most of us totally *identify* with it. When we use the words "I, Me, Mine" that's what we're really referring to. I think, therefore I am. We like to imagine that we're the ones calling the shots.

Yet here we are.

In reality, the subconscious mind is *vastly* more powerful. Sure, you can use your conscious mind to apply discipline and will power, but those efforts are doomed if they contradict the relentless force of habit of your established programming.

Your subconscious pretty much hates change and will do whatever it takes to protect you from it. To protect you from your own *conscious* decision to change and better your life.

Beliefs

If your brain is like a powerful computer, then *beliefs* are the software running it, the code making up your "operating system." And what is a belief? Simply an idea that you have accepted as true, that you no longer question.

An idea like this is relatively impervious to change. Information that contradicts a belief tends to be ignored or dismissed before it can generate uncomfortable cognitive dissonance. Some people get very upset when their beliefs are questioned!

Our beliefs strongly affect the way we perceive what's happening around us. We see what we expect to see. And sometimes there's a kind of satisfaction in that. Being right is comforting. Even when a negative belief seems confirmed through some bad experience, there can be a bitter pleasure in saying "I *knew* it!"

So where do our beliefs come from? Most of them get scooped up in that massive pre-seven-years-old download. To be fair, a whole lot of them are super-helpful. We know what utensil to use for soup. We know to be careful crossing a street. We know that people don't like being yelled at.

But sometimes our beliefs are based on faulty or incomplete information, leading to conclusions that are mistaken or even wrong. And if they're negative and limiting, our beliefs can be enormously counterproductive. For example, believing that you're unlovable is going to make life *so* much harder. Believing that it's never safe to relax will likely burn out your adrenals.

EFT, by the way, is an absolute game changer when it comes to releasing negative, limiting, false beliefs. I'm so excited to share it with you in the next chapter!

The Freeze Response

Interestingly, our worst beliefs tend to come from one particular kind of experience where they get supercharged with strong negative emotion.

You're probably aware of Fight or Flight, that primitive biological reaction when we're attacked or threatened. Adrenaline shoots into our bloodstream, which then gets shunted to our arms and legs. Massive amounts of energy are activated to help us run away or do battle. This is a deeply subconscious program that kicks in instantly, to keep us out of the tiger's belly.

But sometimes we're powerless to run away or fight back. Or we may just feel that way. When we experience helplessness in the face of a threat and Fight or Flight is just *not* an option, our brain flips over to the totally opposite reaction, the Freeze Response.

Instead of activating our energy, Freeze puts us in a state of involuntary relaxation. It's pretty much like going into shock, in the medical sense. We're basically anaesthetized. We go numb, protected from the intensity of the experience by dissociation. This is the basis of trauma.

If you think about it, small children are especially prone to this experience. So much is new to them, and sometimes even benign situations, if they're unexpected, register as threatening. And of course, being so small, children really can't run away or fight back.

You might be thinking: "Oh, but I had a wonderful childhood! Nothing bad happened to me. What does this have to do with my weight?" What's traumatic for a child might seem trivial to an adult.

Have you ever seen terrified little kids having their picture taken with the "Easter Bunny" (an adult in a creepy costume). This big monster has grabbed them, won't let them go, all while their parents are standing by laughing instead of rescuing them. Complete and total Freeze Response trauma.

Why is this relevant?

Time stops when we go into Freeze, and a part of us splits off in that moment.

Our brain assumes we're about to die, so if by some chance we actually survive the experience, it wants us to never forget what happened. Just in case anything like that ever happens again, we'll need to be prepared. So this experience is given super-ultra-top-priority.

That means the entire thing – sights, sounds, smells, tastes, feelings – every bit of it is scooped up and stored in a special kind of memory bank. It's the same place where knowing how to ride a bike is kept.

Did *you* ever learn to ride a bike? If so, you probably know that even if you haven't been on a bike for years and years, barring a head injury, stroke, or some other major damage, you'd still be able to get back on and ride, right? Everyone knows that.

Here's the thing though, that's not because you'd remember how to ride a bike. It's because *you never forgot*. That kind of knowledge is kept current, always ready for instant retrieval. And it's exactly the same for our Freeze Response memories.

It's true that these experiences are encapsulated by dissociation, which protects us from the raw emotional intensity. They may even be pushed down below the level of awareness to the point of amnesia about the incident. But they're always right there, just below the surface, ready to be triggered.

These memories never fade over time. Time may heal all wounds, but our Freeze Response memories are timeless. Without EFT or some other deep intervention that can reach the emotional brain, these memories never heal.

This can be a serious problem. When something going on now just happens to match a detail from one of these encapsulated Freeze Response memories, the dissociation can be breached and suddenly all of the Younger Self's feelings come flooding into *our* body in the here and now. Feelings that are totally out of proportion to our current situation. Sometimes with no obvious reference whatsoever.

When this happens, we can get emotionally hijacked by anxiety, shame, deep sadness or guilt, without even knowing why.

Decisions, Decisions

When we find ourselves in some terrible situation, it's just human nature to ask "Why is this happening to me?" And our answer to that question is basically a decision. A decision about ourselves, or about how life works.

Decisions about ourselves:

> Younger Selves often decide they're unlovable or stupid or unworthy or bad. That they don't deserve love and care. Something along those lines.

> As children we tend to unfairly blame ourselves for anything bad going on. It's rarely true, but we're desperate for some sense of control, some possibility of making things okay.

> For example, Mommy and Daddy are fighting. If I decide it's my fault then maybe I can change what's wrong with me and we'll have a happy family. Even though it's really not my fault, now at least I have hope.

Decisions about the world:

> Or sometimes they'll make a decision about life: the world is a dangerous place. You can't trust anyone. There's never enough to go around. If something good happens, watch out because the other shoe is going to drop.

> The big problem here is that little kids tend to overgeneralize. Instead of deciding not to trust their stepdad (which might actually be a really helpful decision), a child might decide that *all* men

are untrustworthy. Not good! If they're all bad, the child is unlikely to develop discernment.

These decisions we make become beliefs that tend to mess up our lives. In Chapter 16, I've put together a list of negative limiting beliefs specifically related to weight loss, along with an exercise to tap them away.

But there's another aspect to the Freeze Response I want to share here. It's crucial to getting the most from this book.

Younger Selves

When the Freeze Response hits, a part of us splits off and gets trapped, endlessly reliving the bad experience within a capsule of dissociation. I call this split off part a Younger Self, and you probably have *lots* of them. They're an exact holographic replica of who you were in that moment, never growing or changing, until you go back to bust them out of hell.

Although most of the Secret Reasons that keep you from losing weight come from the decisions of your Younger Selves, and it's actually *their* emotional intensity and decisions keeping you stuck, they are NOT your enemy. They are not trying to sabotage you. In fact, they aren't really aware that you even exist. But *helping* them can massively change your life for the better.

In the next chapter you'll find a crash course in EFT tapping, the Super Tool that will empower you to help yourself and these Younger Selves. EFT will get your subconscious back on task to help you attain and maintain your ideal weight.

CHAPTER 3

EFT Crash Course

A re you ready to learn our primary healing Super Tool? The "basic recipe" for EFT tapping is so easy children can learn to do it. At the same time, there's really no limit to how deep you can go with this amazing technique for inner transformation.

In this chapter there's nothing specific to weight; rather I'm giving you the nuts and bolts of the technique here. You can actually use EFT on pretty much anything – money, relationships, health, lost car keys, social anxiety, you name it! We'll be using it to resolve weight issues throughout the rest of the book.

Below are simple written instructions along with a Tapping Points Chart you can download. There's also a link to a helpful how-to video. If you've never experienced EFT, don't worry about getting it right, it's very forgiving. You may be surprised at how well it works right out of the gate!

We'll begin on the next page.

The Basic Recipe

Here's EFT in five simple steps:

1. State the problem (be as specific as you can).

2. Rate how distressing the problem is from zero to ten.

3. Do a "set-up statement" by tapping on the side of your hand and saying: "Even though I have this problem (whatever it is), I deeply love and completely accept myself."

4. Tap around all the points while stating your problem for each point. Go around again and again until you start to feel better.

5. Re-measure the intensity from zero to ten. If the intensity isn't at zero yet, repeat steps 3-5 until you get as close to zero as you can.

To download and print the tapping point chart below and watch my how-to video click here:
tappingthematrix.com/free-how-to-tap-resources/

EFT Tapping Points

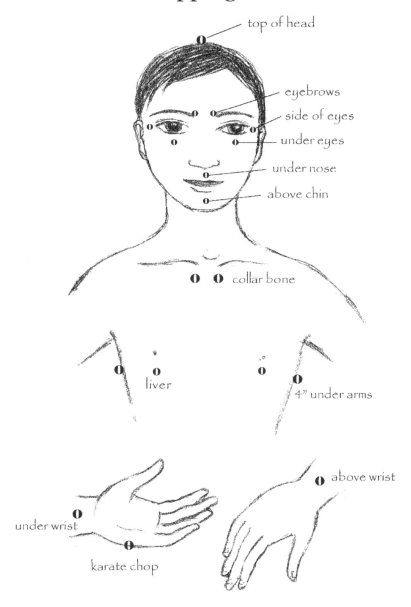

Tapping in Detail

Step 1. State the problem

This is the most important step to get right, which means being as specific as possible. Maybe you're feeling crummy and decide to tap. You could go ahead and tap on "Even though I feel so crummy, I deeply love and completely accept myself." But what does "crummy" actually mean?

It might include being a little sick to your stomach, some anxiety about an upcoming work meeting, feeling resentful that your partner didn't do the dishes last night, plus a twinge of guilt because you still haven't called your mom back and it's been five days.

So "crummy" is really a big tangled ball of yuck. To be most effective with EFT, it's best to tap on one strand at a time. You might do the basic recipe for each thing, and do them one at a time. Or, you could do the whole mess, but make sure and name each strand as you tap through the points.

If you're tapping on a distressing memory, what are the key parts of what happened? And what feelings are coming up? Be sure to name each of these things while tapping on all the specific aspects of the memory.

Step 2. Rate the intensity

With EFT things can change pretty fast. Taking readings as you go is a good way to mark your progress. If the intensity *isn't* going down, or only very slowly, there's a good chance what you're tapping on isn't specific enough.

Our zero to ten scale is often called the "SUD Level" which stands for Subjective Units of Distress (or Discomfort if it's a physical issue). Don't worry about being super accurate with the numbers. Just a guess is good enough.

If you're tapping on an old memory, rate the intensity you're feeling *now*, not at the time it happened.

Step 3. The Set-Up Statement

Tap on the side of your hand below the pinky – the "Karate Chop Point." Either hand is fine.

The Set-Up Statement activates our specific issue in the emotional brain so that the effects of the tapping are targeted. It also lowers resistance to change, at least temporarily. And finally, it balances out the problem with a key affirmation:

"Even though I have this _____, I deeply love and completely accept myself" or

"Even though I have this _____, I choose to forgive myself, as best I can" or

"Even though I have this _____, I want to get to a calm and peaceful place."

Just fill in the _____ with whatever specific problem you'd like to change.

A Set-Up Statement is done before each new "round" of tapping, which usually involves tapping around the points over and over until you feel a shift. The Set-Up Statement for the next round will usually focus on what's left, whatever is still bothering you.

Step 4. Tap through the points

Tap on each point, starting at the top of the head and working your way down your body. We usually tap about 7-10 times on each point, though the exact number isn't important. With each point say a "reminder phrase" to keep the problem activated.

You can simply repeat the same words from your setup statement over and over: "This headache, this headache, this headache, this headache..." but after a while, the words might start to lose their meaning. Better to use descriptive adjectives to be even more specific.

You might say: "This headache, this headache on the right side of my head, this splitting headache, this sharp pain when I move my head too fast, this sharp, stabbing pain on the right side of my head, this headache, this frustrating headache that just won't go away..." And so on.

You don't need a PhD in psychology to know what words to say. Simply describe every aspect of what's wrong as you tap around the points. Even if you do just say the same words over and over, it's still likely to help quite a bit.

You'll notice that some points are on the midline, while others are bilateral. It really doesn't matter whether you tap on both sides or just one or the other. If I have both hands free, I'll usually tap on both sides just because it feels better.

The less you actually think about the act of tapping the better. Ideally, you're mostly focused on the problem at hand. There's no need to stop once you've gone through all the points once. More often we'll go around and around the points in "rounds" until noticing a shift in how we feel.

Step 5. Re-measure the intensity

When you do feel a shift from the tapping, it's time to re-measure your SUD level. Our scale in EFT is zero to ten, and that zero is important. Zero means the problem (or our emotional intensity *about* the problem) is totally gone, which suggests that it's much less likely to come back. Ideally, we tap every issue down to zero.

Sometimes you might have a "better quit while I'm ahead" kind of feeling. If the SUD level drops from 8 to a 3, that feels pretty amazing! So let's not push our luck, right? No! Keep tapping! Get that intensity as close to zero as you can.

Focusing on the Negative

Remember my advice to be specific in Step One? That really means be specific about what's wrong. EFT is all about discharging and sloughing off the old, negative, worn-out stuff that doesn't belong. That means we need to name it!

This can be disconcerting, especially for Law of Attraction devotees. You might have a superstition that saying anything negative will attract it to you. Don't worry! It doesn't work that way with tapping.

If a negative thought isn't already stuck in your subconscious, I guarantee you won't implant it with EFT. The words will just go in one ear and out the other.

On the other hand, if we name something negative that *is* lurking in the subconscious, there's often a little spike in emotional intensity as it's discharged. Even if there's a big spike in intensity, it's always followed by immediate relief – kind of like throwing up if you've eaten something spoiled. You feel so much better once it's out of your system.

Cleaning Out the Wound

Imagine you fell and got a gash in your arm and it's all full of dirt and grime and little bits of gravel. You go to the ER, and a nurse says, "Oh no! That looks pretty bad. Let's get that all wrapped up in some nice sterile bandages."

You might be worried that he skipped a step – and rightly so! Unless he thoroughly cleans out the wound and gets all of that crud out of it, how can it heal? It's way more likely to get infected.

EFT is all about cleaning out the wounds so they can finally heal. Don't be afraid to name, acknowledge and *feel into* the worst of it while tapping. In my workshops, I urge my students to "Go for the jugular!"

That said, it's totally okay to tap on positive statements. There's value in affirming that we love, accept and forgive ourselves. It can be helpful to voice the way we'd like things to change and tap into gratitude. Just don't shy away from clearing out the scary bad stuff too. That's what will really change your life.

A Simple Trick

When you tap on the scripts in this book, you might need to go through them many times to get that SUD level towards zero.

If you're tapping on your own without a script, I highly recommend using a timer. If your mind is anything like mine, it's a slippery devil. I'll start tapping on some issue and suddenly realize I'm looking at Instagram or doing the dishes. How did *that* happen?

These days I just set a timer and keep tapping until it dings. I recommend doing 5 to 8 minutes at a go. Maybe 12 minutes for really difficult issues. Then check the SUD level and do a second round if need be. I've been doing this timer trick for the last few years, and it's made a huge difference for me.

Working with a Practitioner

EFT is a fantastic self-help tool, but sometimes it's best to work with an experienced practitioner. If you're feeling fragile or freaked out, or dealing with severe abuse memories, heavy depression, panic attacks or anything really overwhelming, it's definitely best to get some expert help. Even with "garden variety" life issues, you'll likely make more progress working with someone good.

Take it for a Spin

Are you ready to take EFT for a test drive? Pick an issue you'd like to see change. Go through those 5 simple steps and have a go! Or if you'd like to watch my how-to video first, or download the tapping points chart, here's the link again:

tappingthematrix.com/free-how-to-tap-resources/

In the next chapter I'll share a special way to help your Younger Selves with tapping, to set them free from their Freeze-Response tape loops.

CHAPTER 4

Tapping for Younger Selves

Usually when we're tapping we're focused on something wrong in the here and now. Whether it's negative feelings, physical pain, or some bad situation we're confronted with, we're most often tapping for ourselves in real time.

This is true even when we're tapping on a bad memory. We're discharging whatever feelings we're having here and now about what happened back then.

And because we're working on our own stuff, it just makes sense to use the words *I* and *my* while we're tapping: "Even though *I* have this headache" or "this pain in *my* foot," for example.

That said, most of the Secret Reasons exist because of a Younger Self and *their* feelings and decisions. Thanks to the Freeze Response, it doesn't matter how long ago their trauma happened. As far as your subconscious is concerned, it's happening right now.

So is there a way we can use tapping to help a Younger Self? Yes! We can address our words to them directly, and instead of saying *I* we'll be saying *You* as we tap for them.

As we go through the Secret Reasons you'll find tapping scripts at the end of each chapter. Some chapters have additional scripts specifically for the Younger Self who may be involved.

These scripts attempt to address most of the possible decisions and feelings that *might* be involved, but if any of the words aren't a good match, feel free to skip them, change them to something more apt, or just go ahead and say them anyway – they won't do your Younger Self any harm.

Depending on how well you can tune into your Younger Self, here are two ways to proceed.

Method Number One

Use this approach if you only have a vague or general idea of what might have happened, and it's hard to visualize your Younger Self. You might only have a somewhat abstract sense of her.

Simply tap on yourself, but begin addressing the words to this imaginary child. Just use your imagination as best you can and say the words as if you were addressing any child about her age.

Remember, for you it's a memory, but for them it's a current event!

For example:

"Even though this terrible thing has happened, I want you to know you're safe, it's not your fault and you're not alone, I'm here to help you..."

We have two main purposes here: a) discharge the Younger Self's shock and emotional intensity, and b) help them change their mind about *why* the bad thing is happening. It's especially important, for our purposes, to help them let go of any notion that carrying extra weight is a great idea.

Method Number Two

If you *do* have a clear image of your Younger Self – if she's so real you could just reach out and tap on her, that's awesome! And that's exactly what I'd like you to imagine.

By that, I mean *picture* that you're tapping on her, while tapping the same EFT points on your own body. Start with the set-up statement on her karate chop point, then move to the top of her head and around through all of the points on her face and body.

Ideally, tap on your own body with one hand, while picturing that you're tapping on your Younger Self with the other hand. If you need help visualizing, try tapping in the air where your Younger Self is standing or sitting.

For some people, tapping on themselves distracts too much from picturing the tapping on their Younger Self. One workaround is to simply tap on your own collarbone point, while doing all the points on your Younger Self. Or just skip tapping on yourself altogether.

Tapping on the Younger Self is definitely the most important thing here, and while you tap you'll be addressing the words to them, out loud or silently in your own mind.

For example:

"Even though you're so scared right now, you're not alone, I've come back to help you..."

Before you start tapping, it might be helpful to imagine introducing yourself, something like: "Hi there, I'm *you* from the future, all grown up! I've come back to help you."

It can also be *very* helpful to imagine freezing the scene and everyone else in the picture just like a statue. That way any danger or drama is stopped and you're more likely to get your Younger Self's full attention.

At that point you can start reading from the Younger Self script. Or if you have a really good connection, try asking her what she's feeling and simply tap on what she tells you, adding any reassurance you'd like to give her.

As you go through the tapping, your Younger Self should start feeling better and better. And because she's actually a split off part of you, you'll probably feel her relief register in your own body.

You'll soon have a chance to try this, once we get to the Secret Reasons section of the book. First though, let's take a look at how cultural programming may have set the stage for your weight issues.

CHAPTER 5

Cultural Programming

H ow do you know if you're good-looking enough?

Is it possible that the way you regard yourself, and especially your body, might be influenced by television, movies, magazines and social media? If so, how strong *is* that influence, and do you think it might be a problem?

Growing up in a family teaches us most of what we know about how to live, but when I was growing up most families spent a lot of time sitting around the TV. Now we're all just sitting around looking at our phones.

There's no denying that most of us are bombarded by an endless stream of images, programming and ideals. And that stream isn't just random. The media we take in has been carefully crafted to affect our behavior.

I know it seems like there's a huge diversity of media outlets, providing an incredibly wide array of content, but at the time of this writing, just six corporations own at least 90% of all media channels. And *all* of their content, across *all* of the many platforms, is carefully coordinated and has been for decades.

This includes movies, TV, magazines, scientific publications, the fashion industry, pop stars and celebrities. Even many social media influencers have corporate sponsorship.

Why is this relevant? There are hidden agendas behind all of this coordination that may have set you up for weight loss obsession. I'd be negligent not to mention it, even at the risk of sounding like a crazy conspiracy theorist.

The crazy conspiracy I want to focus on here is the agenda to shatter your self-esteem just to pick your pocket. Especially if you're a woman. When I was a little kid in the 60s, the female ideal began to shift from Marilyn Monroe to Twiggy. From full figured womanly to pixie boyishness. Around the same time, advertising began transitioning to an ideal of youth – from mature adult to teenager.

Unobtainable

I was born in 1959 and raised in the United States. Over the years, the media mono-culture I grew up in has massively diversified. Barbie and the Marlboro Man have been joined by any number of multicultural icons. But is anyone any happier?

Across all channels, we're *still* presented with ideals or standards of beauty that are simply unobtainable, and this is by design. Call me cynical, but fostering dissatisfaction, envy, insecurity and desperation is a winning strategy for advertisers. It moves a lot of product.

While there are plenty of other physical opportunities for insecurity and low self-esteem – hair, skin, breast size, hygiene, fashionability, and status symbols, I do believe fat reigns supreme. The weight-industrial complex is in a league of its own, cranking out endless products and programs that promise the moon but rarely deliver permanent results.

It's the perfect scam, really. If you don't lose weight with the latest fad diet or superfood or exercise regime, it's always your own fault. *You* failed somehow. You didn't stick with it long enough; you didn't have enough discipline. *You* failed, not the program.

True story: I put off writing this book for years out of reluctance to be associated with the unethical grifters taking advantage of people's weight loss suffering. Perhaps the promises I'm making sound just as "too good to be true"? I really hope not! My sincere intention is to empower you with the tools to effect real and lasting change for the better!

What's Your Motivation?

I've worked with a lot of clients, mostly women, who seriously wanted to lose weight. But not all for the same reasons. For some, the motivation was purely aesthetic. Falling short of their ideal appearance was absolutely intolerable for them. For others, it was more a matter of freedom of movement, in the physical sense. They felt like they were wearing a fat suit that slowed them down and made dancing or yoga or hiking a lot less enjoyable.

Yet another motivation might have been wanting more respect or seeking an upgrade in the attention they were getting. Let's face it, there's still a lot of fat-shaming in some areas. Losing weight may seem like a necessary achievement for having better self-esteem.

I've also had a few clients whose obesity had reached the point where serious health risks were demanding immediate attention. Aside from debilitating mobility issues, the threats of heart disease, stroke and diabetes were no joke at all.

Whatever *your* motivation, I'm hoping to help you to reach your ideal weight and stay there. My own ideal for this process is ever-increasing health and vitality. I see that as a worthy goal, in and of itself.

I believe there's an important difference between "Pretty" and "Beautiful." I think of *pretty* as being both superficial and ephemeral. It tends to fade as we grow older. Beauty, on the other hand, comes from health, happiness and a loving heart. More than skin deep, it's something that radiates from within and can definitely grow as we age.

Losing weight is really about feeling more and more at home in your own body. Losing the Secret Reasons will make you happier, more loving and thus, more beautiful.

Fat as the Enemy

I know that other countries, and certain subcultures here in the US, may have wildly different standards of health and beauty. For some, carrying extra weight or being super curvy may be highly prized or desirable. Since you're reading this book though, I'm guessing that's not the kind of culture you find yourself in.

For the last 50 years or so, fat has been demonized, at least here in the US. As you may be aware, people seen as overweight or fat have been denigrated, made the butt of jokes and seen as fair game for bullies. Carrying extra weight meant you were considered less attractive, taken less seriously, and were valued less than thin or fit people. Expectations were lower, as were opportunities.

Even a person who carries extra pounds but feels okay about themselves, may still get a lot of shit from other people. With all of that in mind, do you think this may have affected your sense of what you should weigh?

Ideal Weight

The concept of an Ideal Body Weight based on height, age and gender has been around for a long time. Doctors have come up with competing formulas, but put together they provide a basic accepted range.

I'm not sure whether that has much bearing for most of my clients. If they have a specific weight in mind, it's more often based on their personal history than what some doctor or website suggests. They might want to get back to what they weighed in their early 20s, for example.

In working your way through this book, I hope you won't be compulsively checking the bathroom scale. That's definitely counterproductive. I suppose if you just can't help it, at least do some tapping while you're checking!

That said, having some sort of ideal number in mind might actually be helpful as a goal. We're all about working *with* your subconscious, so let's give it a numerical suggestion for recalibrating your appetite and metabolism. And if that number happens to be healthy for your body, fantastic!

Obtainability

Sadly, I've seen clients and loved ones become attached to an aesthetic standard that's simply unobtainable for them. No doubt that's a win for media programming, creating a customer for life, but for that person it's a recipe for misery and failure.

Years ago, I worked with a wonderful Māori woman in New Zealand. As a people, the Māori tend to be pretty big, but my client had grown up thinking she should look like her Barbie doll! No joke. Tapping away that artificial standard gave her a new freedom to appreciate her own beauty.

If *your* template for ideal weight came from the pages of Vogue magazine, endless TV shows and movies, or skinny Instagram influencers half your age, could it be that you've been sold a bill of goods? One that's not in your own best interest? I'm not telling you to totally scrap your aesthetic ideal, but if it's more pretty than beautiful, and especially if it seems unobtainable, I do suggest taking a good hard look.

This book is about helping you achieve more and more freedom. Freedom from the past. And freedom to become your best and most authentic self. Whatever number you've chosen for an ideal weight, it may change as you change. It's all good.

In the next chapter we'll tackle what may be the most important freedom of all – freedom from self-loathing.

CHAPTER 6

Self-Loathing

With a new weight-issue client, the first thing I do is ask for their "self-loathing index." In other words, on a scale of zero to ten, how bad do they feel about themselves?

Often there are two levels to this. Sometimes they just really hate their body and the way they look. Sometimes there's something specific – it might be the fat on their belly or the underside of their arms. Or maybe they're disgusted by lumpy cellulite, or think their butt is too big.

On an entirely different level, some of my clients hate themselves for being undisciplined or weak. Being "fat" means their failure is terribly public. In their mind, everyone can see they have no self-control and thinks they're a loser. For them, carrying extra weight feels extremely humiliating.

How About You?

Let me ask you to go ahead and rate your own self-loathing, zero to ten. Whether it's because of how you look, that you even have a weight issue at all, or it's one all-inclusive bundle of hating on yourself, what would you say?

As you may have guessed, I do have an agenda here. I'd like to help you tap down *your* number as low as possible. In fact, I'd really like your level of self-loathing to drop all the way down to zero. Why? Because it's an essential first step in getting you the results you want so badly.

Lucky for us, radical self-acceptance is actually baked into the EFT setup statement, right? "I deeply love and completely *accept* myself."

Some of my clients are really resistant to this idea, at least in the beginning. I get it. If you're consumed with disgust of your own body, then self-acceptance is probably the *last* thing you'd want. What a terrible idea! Rudimentary logic suggests that if you accept yourself the way you are right now, you'll lose your motivation to change. And that's not okay!

On the surface this may seem legit. It just makes sense, right? But let me ask you this: how is *not* accepting yourself, in fact LOATHING yourself, working out for you? Not so well I guess, or you wouldn't be reading this book.

The Paradox

If you were going to hate yourself into becoming thin, wouldn't that have worked by now? Like maybe a long time ago? If hating yourself thin was an effective strategy, there'd be a lot of very thin, miserable people walking around.

I'll admit that some people *are* able to use self-hatred as a motivator. They force themselves to diet and exercise. Perhaps they do lose weight but the pounds almost always come back and then some. Why is this?

What if self-loathing actually *drives* your overeating? What if that sense of disgust or despair about your body actually increases your need for comfort which leads to craving and overindulging in "comfort food"?

There is a strange paradox at work here. For any kind of real and lasting change to happen, you have to let go of the emotional intensity of self-loathing. You have to love and accept your body just as it is right now *before* you can truly attain the body you desire.

Consider this possibility: that your body is a perfect reflection of your emotional state.

If this is true (and I believe that it is), then changing your emotional state is the *only* thing that will bring about deep, lasting change. Ugly emotions will never create a beautiful physical body.

Your Faithful Servant

Beyond being a reflection of your emotional state, your body is also your faithful servant. You probably don't remember, but your Younger Self *asked* it to hold onto fat as some kind of protection. That's what the Secret Reasons are all about.

Here's the Truth: your body doesn't *want* to carry extra weight; it's a burden. Your body is actually doing you a favor. As soon as your Younger Self stops asking or "needing" that extra fat, your body will be absolutely delighted to reset to its ideal healthy weight. It really *is* on your side.

Once they realize the truth of this, some of my clients actually feel guilty for being so mean and hateful toward their own body. It's so unfair! It really is a sobering realization that your body has been doing you a favor. But let's not entertain any more guilt.

The more you love, accept and forgive yourself, the happier and lighter your body will become. Happier equals lighter.

In the next section, we'll explore and begin to resolve the Secret Reasons one by one. Before we move on though, let's tackle this not-so-secret issue of self-loathing head on with an EFT tapping script – the first of many we'll be using in this book.

Since this is our first tapping script, here are some suggestions and helpful things to know.

Tapping with a Script

Much like the script an actor reads for a movie or play, I've put together lines for you to read while tapping. These scripts are intended to bring up negative thoughts and feelings so that your tapping can work its magic and take away their charge.

You'll notice there are many lines in the script, some shorter, some longer. Each time you move to a new tapping point, just read the next line – one complete line for each point. And just keep moving through the points.

The scripts in this book may include words and ideas that don't really fit for you, or don't seem to apply, and that's okay. Some of these lines will probably resonate strongly for you while others won't. You can just skip those lines, or read them anyway – it won't do any harm. It's impossible to implant negative ideas into your subconscious this way.

It's important to know this because some of the scripts include extreme, absurd, ludicrous and outrageous statements! Things that you would never allow yourself to think or feel consciously. You may even hate saying the words.

The thing is, we're really trying to help your *subconscious* mind, which may be harboring all kinds of dark, yucky and primitive stuff. Giving voice to such extreme or absurd statements *while tapping* is a good way of releasing this unhealthy junk *if* it happens to be there.

So please just go ahead and read the outrageous bits. As long as you're tapping it won't do any harm and may actually do a surprising amount of good.

If there are particular lines that trigger you or have a strong negative emotional charge, it's probably a great idea to repeat those lines a number of times!

If possible, I suggest reading the words aloud, and allow yourself to read them with feeling. That's a bit more powerful than just reading them silently in your head. But don't let a lack of privacy stop you! Silently in your head will work too.

Please do NOT just read the words without also tapping. That would be useless at best, and might even be counterproductive. Remember, EFT is about discharging, sloughing off and releasing old junk that's been stuck. The scripts focus on negative yucky stuff, since that's what we're getting rid of.

Let me say it again, please do *not* read the scripts without also tapping.

You'll almost certainly need to tap through the scripts multiple times. Especially if your emotional intensity level starts off pretty high. You might even notice yourself becoming *more* upset as you go – don't worry, just keep tapping. That intensification sometimes happens before a massive release.

Ideally, we're trying to tap that level down to zero, or as close to zero as possible. Once you can read the words and there's no real feeling at all, you're free!

DIY

One problem with tapping scripts is that they're necessarily a one-size-fits-all approach, and unavoidably generic. That's why writing your own script might be a powerful option, if you're so inspired. You can make it specific to *all* of the particular things you hate about your body and hate about yourself...let it rip!

Do-it-yourself customized scripts are almost always better, but I do have high hopes that the ones included in this book will do the trick for you.

Note: If you somehow skipped the how-to-tap chapter, better stop here and go back and read it first.

Tapping for Self-Loathing

Tapping on the karate chop point:

Even though I'm so fat and disgusting and too undisciplined to lose weight, I choose to love and accept myself as best I can.

Tapping through the points:

I hate my body
I hate the way it looks
I'm so gross
So ugly
When I look in the mirror I want to throw up
I have all of this fat
I can't stand it
I can't stand myself for being this way
All of this self-hate

I have no excuse
I did this to myself
I'm so weak
I have no willpower

Everyone can see what a failure I am
I can't hide it
It's so embarrassing being seen like this
I'm so ashamed

All of this self-loathing
This disgust with myself
My big fat stomach
My fat arms
I hate myself for looking this way
I hate myself for getting so fat
I hate myself for being so weak
For eating all the wrong stuff
I'm such a weak-willed failure
And everyone can see it
This feeling of shame
This self-hate

I absolutely HATE my body right now
It's so gross
So disgusting
All of this disgusting blubber
All of this disgusting fat on my body
I've tried so hard to lose weight and I always fail
Everyone can see what a failure I am
I just hate myself so much

I'm too fat and I can't change it
Nothing I try works
I can't diet successfully
I can't lose the weight and keep it off
It feels so hopeless and I *hate* it
I hate myself
And I hate my body for being so fat
All of this stress around being too fat
All of this self-hate and self-loathing

But my poor body is working so hard to protect me
I'm a sensitive person and sometimes life is too hard

There's so much stress in my life
And I'm carrying so much stress from the past
Maybe my body really is trying to protect me with all this extra fat
Maybe all this fat is insulation,
Insulation my body is creating to protect me

I want to let go of all this stress
So my body won't *have* to protect me anymore
I want to let it have a vacation
I want to let it have time off from all the stress and fear
All this distress
All these hard old feelings
All this sadness and fear and anger and shame

I want to tap this all away so my body can just relax
My current weight sucks
But maybe it really is a perfect match for my emotional state
And I choose to change that state
I choose to start by loving and accepting my body just the way it is right now
I don't like the way I look
I don't like the way I move in the world
I'm too heavy
I'm too fat

But I choose to love and appreciate my body as best I can
Even though I don't like the way it's trying to protect me
I want to get to a place of gratitude
I want to get to a better emotional state
My body can't help but shed the weight gracefully, effortlessly
As my emotional state lightens up my body will lighten up too
Without any kind of struggle
My body is my ally, not my enemy

I choose to see it as my patient friend and loyal servant

I forgive myself for hating my body and choose to see it in
a new way
I choose to feel hopeful and optimistic that I really *can*
shed the old distress
The old emotional hurt that I needed to be protected from
I'm going to get to an entirely new place in my life
And I thank my body for all its hard work and for
protecting me
I choose to love and accept myself just as I am right now
And as I am changing

*Check your emotional intensity (SUD level) and go back
through the script again until you get it down to zero*

The Seven Secret Reasons

The more we reject our own Younger Selves (that part of us that misbehaves), the more we condemn them, push them away and try to create distance, the more autonomous they become. This shows up as out-of-control compulsive behavior – not good!

Helping your Younger-Selves can massively change your life for the better.

CHAPTER 7

Binge Eating

Ginny came to me for help with binge eating, which had become a nightly torment for her. Retired now, she'd had a successful career, a reasonably good marriage, and overall, life was really not very stressful. Except for the binge eating, which left her feeling absolutely devastated, hopeless and physically sick.

It made absolutely no sense to her why this was happening. The urge to binge would come on every night after her husband had gone to bed. It made no difference that she'd had dinner, that she wasn't hungry, that she'd told herself "Not again! Not tonight!" The compulsion was overwhelming and she'd end up ferociously cramming food into her mouth like a starving wolf.

What do you suppose causes binge eating like this? Is it because food is yummy? Is it because the person is just weak-willed? No and no. Ginny wasn't enjoying the food at all; it was a nightmare to her. As for being weak, why is there a struggle in the first place?

Reenactment of Feelings

The key to this mystery lies in the compulsion. Where did it come from? What's it all about, really? And most importantly, how do we turn it off? In Ginny's case, we used tapping to find the answers, and what emerged might surprise you.

With EFT it's usually best to start with whatever bad feelings are strongest, in this case it was hopelessness and devastation. As we began tapping the intensity down for those feelings, something new and rather excruciating came up for Ginny – a terrible kind of shame at having failed yet again.

At first, confronting this shame was almost unbearable for her, but the tapping did its magic and after quite a few rounds the intensity melted away, making room for new clarity. I asked Ginny, "When is the first time you felt this same feeling of shame?" Immediately a memory surfaced for her.

When Ginny was in second grade, her class was learning to tell time. This was before digital clocks, so you had to look at the hands to figure it out. Though her best friend said "This is easy," Ginny was baffled. She was a smart girl, and was used to doing well in school, but even though she worked on the homework that night, she just couldn't seem to crack the code.

To make matters worse, the next day the teacher actually called on Ginny to stand up and answer a time-telling question in front of the class. As she stood there stammering, feeling like a total failure, her classmates began to snicker and laugh at her. No doubt the teacher scolded them, but the damage was done, and Ginny imagined the teacher herself was full of contempt.

As adults, it's easy to be dismissive of such childhood traumas. They may even seem comical to us now. But for Ginny's seven-year-old Younger Self, she was trapped in a searing *agony* of shame over her failure. This was an especially bad Freeze Response moment.

You might be wondering, what does any of that have to do with Ginny's binge eating now? How could a problem telling time be related to food and overeating? Remember, it's the *compulsion* that holds the key.

Trauma Capsules

In Chapter 1 we looked at how the Freeze Response encapsulates a traumatic moment with dissociation. This protects us from the raw intensity of the feelings – in this case the terrible shame Ginny's seven-year-old Younger Self was feeling. Time gets frozen for that Younger Self and they're trapped, endlessly reliving the terrible event.

This process of encapsulation is beautifully described by neuro-physician Dr. Robert Scaer, who coined the term "trauma capsule." His book *8 Keys to Brain Body Balance* is highly recommended.

Sometimes the Younger Selves in these "trauma capsules" get triggered by current events (for example, our decision to go on a diet). Their feelings can come flooding into us. But what was going on with Ginny was a bit different.

If you think about it, these encapsulated moments are much like an actual cyst, where something toxic gets all sealed up, to isolate it from the rest of the body. In this case, the toxic thing is the intense negative feelings of the Younger Self, sealed off so we can get on with life.

The thing is, our subconscious mind really hates our "trauma capsules," and wants to get them out of our system. And no wonder – whenever we get "triggered" these capsules can leak, and that's dangerous. Also, it takes energy to keep them sealed up. The more intense the feelings, the more energy required. They're a drain on our system. So yeah, the subconscious wants them gone. What a good idea!

But there's a problem. A really big problem. There's zero creative intelligence in the subconscious. There's no one home, so to speak, so no chance of coming up with a new strategy. The *only* thing the subconscious can do is reenact what's been done already. Repeat, redo, replay, reenact – it's a one-trick pony. However, it's really quite good at that one trick of repetition.

Lather, Rinse, Repeat

So what happens is this: In an attempt to heal us, our powerful yet completely uncreative subconscious mind sets us up to have the same awful experiences over and over.

That might mean the same sort of bully shows up in your life, again and again. Maybe the first one was in middle school and the latest was your last boss. That's your subconscious at work.

Or maybe you have a friend who keeps getting together with the same sort of deadbeat guy. She's currently supporting her third worthless husband. She doesn't realize these guys are actually a stand-in for her dad when she was a traumatized little girl.

In Ginny's case, her subconscious seemed hell-bent on reenacting that searing shame in 2nd grade. Only now, instead of failing to tell time, she was failing to control her bingeing. Very different circumstances, but the emotion was weirdly the same.

You might be thinking, why on Earth would anyone *want* to re-experience horrible situations or feelings like that? They don't! That's the last thing they want. But it's a compulsion, right? That means their subconscious mind is in charge. Not only that, their subconscious has made healing their trauma (through reenactment) a top priority!

Unfortunately, this is pretty much the worst strategy of all time! Instead of healing us, instead of actually resolving the original trauma, repetition just keeps digging the hole deeper. The negative feelings become more and more familiar, and our negative beliefs are reinforced.

Sometimes it may feel like fate, like we're cursed, because the bad thing keeps happening to us and we're helpless to avoid it.

The Grand Opening

Any time my client has compulsive, self-destructive behavior, whether it's binge eating or something else, I'm always curious to see if it's a reenactment of negative feelings. Like Ginny, are they being dragged through hell again and again just because some Younger Self is trapped and suffering, while the subconscious is trying to fix things?

I realize this is a totally counter-intuitive way to look at things. It makes no rational sense why anyone would put themselves through crippling shame, or rage, or feeling powerlessness, or whatever. But honestly, there's nothing rational about the subconscious mind. All it knows how to do is repeat, redo, revisit, reenact.

Just to be clear, I'm not saying this is the *only* cause of compulsive behavior. There could be other things going on. But reenactment is definitely worth looking into.

For example, I think it's safe to say that no one ever feels good after binge eating. Along with feeling physically yucky, there may be feelings of shame, despair, rage, failure, being out of control, or all of the above. For everyone I've worked with, it's a pretty miserable experience.

So, the question we need to ask is this: If we're having a recurring Shit Show, when was the Grand Opening? Which Younger Self first felt these feelings and why? Finding her, and helping her for real, will probably shut down the whole reenactment machine.

With Ginny, once that 2nd grade memory surfaced, we were able to tap on all the related feelings, essentially helping her Younger Self let go of all the shame, embarrassment, sense of failure and being exposed. Once Ginny was able to remember the event with zero emotional charge, the compulsion was gone and didn't come back.

How do I know it was gone? Well, that's the one good thing about having a binge eating issue. Maybe the only good thing. You know when it's over. That night Ginny must have been on pins and needles (she didn't tell me that part, but I'm guessing). But she did say there was no urge to binge whatsoever. Not even for a little bedtime snack.

Even if you can't trace a compulsion back to its original trauma, just tapping on the intense negative feelings may be enough to shut the whole thing down. Especially if you can get the SUD level down to zero.

In our next chapter we'll take a look at one of the strongest of all the Secret Reasons, protection from sexual attention. But first here's a tapping script for compulsive reenactment of negative feelings, focusing on binge eating and shame. Feel free to modify it for other compulsive behaviors and feelings.

Tapping for Binge Eating

Tapping on your karate chop point:

Even though I can't control myself and end up feeling all of this shame, I choose to love and accept myself as best I can.

Tapping through the points:

All of this shame
I should be able to control myself
But I can't
I can't make myself stop

I tell myself to stop but it doesn't work
I'm totally out of control
I can't stop eating until I'm totally sick
It's so disgusting
So shameful
I just can't stand it

All of this shame
This terrible feeling of being out of control
All this shame
This feeling of failure
Failure to control myself
I'm so undisciplined
Such a loser
I can't even stop myself
It just feels so degrading
I should be better than this
I should have control
I should be able to stop
I shouldn't even start in the first place

But I still choose to forgive myself as best I can
If I met another person with this bingeing problem
Would I judge them the way I judge myself?
So harshly?
Or would I feel some kind of compassion?
Would I wonder what happened to them?
I choose to give myself the same compassion I'd give any
other person
Something must have happened to *me*

It's just too overwhelming
All of this shame
I don't want anyone to know I do this
It's so embarrassing
So shameful

But what if I refuse to feel ashamed?
What if the shame is actually making it worse?

What if compassion for myself would make it stop?
God, I want it to stop so bad!
It's so degrading, so horrible
I can't believe I'm so out of control
But what if?
What if the whole point of this bingeing is to feel shame?
What if my brain is looking for an excuse to feel the
shame that was already there?
It's gross and disgusting what I've been doing
But what if I can forgive myself?
What if I just *refuse* to judge myself?
Refuse to feel that ugly shame?

This compulsion
This compulsion to binge
Even when I'm not hungry
Even when I feel sick
I just can't stop cramming food into my face
I can't get enough in me fast enough
What if the whole point is to feel all this shame?
What if I refuse to play along?
What if I really can stop feeling all this shame?

When I get the flu I might throw up
And that's totally gross
But I don't judge myself
I'm just sick and couldn't help it
I might feel really sorry for myself for throwing up
But not this horrible self-hate
What if I can find some compassion for myself?
The same compassion I'd give a total stranger?
I *choose* to forgive myself
I choose to forgive myself for having this problem
For having this embarrassing binge eating problem

Even if I never get over it,
I choose to love and accept myself
As best I can
If I was going to shame it away,

it would have happened by now
If I could hate myself free, I'd be free already
Even if I don't *deserve* to love and accept myself
I choose to love and accept myself anyway
Even if loving and accepting myself doesn't work
Even if it doesn't stop it
Even if I *keep* bingeing
I still want to feel good about who I am
I want to feel good about my life
And I deeply love and completely accept myself

Please check in with your SUD level. If there's more intensity, keep tapping through the script to get it as close to zero as possible.

CHAPTER 8

Protection from Sexual Attention

Note: If you have unresolved sexual trauma and find this chapter triggering, I suggest you stop and seek out professional help with a practitioner skilled in resolving sexual abuse trauma.

Sadly, unwanted sexual attention is far and away the most common Secret Reason for being (and staying) overweight, at least for the clients I've worked with. Especially when that unwanted attention led to actual abuse.

Sexual abuse, especially of children, is a hidden epidemic that goes back at least to Victorian times when Sigmund Freud was investigating "hysteria" among young women in upper-class Vienna. He made the shocking discovery that many of his hysteria patients had been molested by their fathers or uncles.

Freud discovered that encouraging his patients to talk about their traumas while attentively listening sometimes had a major impact on their well-being. His "talking cure" set the stage for modern psychotherapy. This was back in the 1890s.

Today, with EFT tapping, we now have ways to more thoroughly resolve and heal from these traumas. Before we jump in though, I should mention that with any really intense trauma, it's always best to work with a skilled practitioner. Especially those trained in advanced EFT work such as Hacking Reality or Matrix Reimprinting.

My goal for this chapter is to explore what might be going on for you with this Secret Reason, especially regarding weight issues, and hopefully take enough of the charge off to give you the freedom to change.

Becoming Un-Attractive

Putting on excess weight to become unattractive to sexual predation is a subconscious strategy that can be so emotionally charged, it can override even serious life-threatening health concerns.

If *you've* experienced sexual trauma, whether molestation, incest, rape or even just creepy attention, you'll almost certainly have at least one Younger Self trapped in the endless tape loop of that terrible experience.

The two most important aspects for us to address here are the raw emotions of these Younger Selves and what decisions they made about themselves or about the world in that moment of great distress.

We'll do some tapping at the end of this chapter that will hopefully be helpful, but first let's explore some of the various complicating factors.

For my clients, the most common age when unwanted attention first happens is around puberty, when their body begins developing sexually. That said, sexual abuse can happen at any age, from infancy on up.

Generally speaking, the younger we are when sexual abuse begins, the more *foundational* the damage to our identity, our trust in life and other people, and our sense of safety in the world. It's possible to actually dissociate somewhat from our own body or sexualized body parts.

I've had clients who, as young children, were bribed with treats to go along with abuse or to allow it to happen. This can set up a very complicated, shame-based relationship with food and eating, especially when it comes to any kind of treat.

When unwanted attention begins around the time of puberty, putting on excess weight may be a way of blurring the sexual changes and becoming less "shapely."

With enough fat the waist disappears and breasts may be de-emphasized. Resemblance to youthful models, glamorous actresses or sexualized celebrities is diminished. At least that's the plan. If a decision was made by the Younger Self that sexual attention is dangerous and to be avoided at all costs, then what a huge relief that extra weight must bring.

Ironically, the strategy of putting on weight doesn't always work, at least in the sense of becoming invisible to perpetrators. Yet it does work to make us FEEL unattractive, which has the effect of dampening our own youthful exuberance and naïve confidence.

We're much less likely to slip up and accidentally act "sexy" if we use fat as an excuse to feel gross and disgusting. Feeling ugly may become strongly linked with the all-important sense of safety.

What's Love Got to Do with It?

Another issue that tends to show up around the time of puberty is excruciating self-consciousness and social anxiety. As our body becomes increasingly sexual, there can be intensifying pressure to engage in romantic relationships. This doesn't always go well!

Quite apart from any sexual intrusion, feelings of romantic rejection and humiliation can be incredibly traumatic.

As adults we may be inclined to minimize this, passing it off as an awkward but amusing stage we went through that's good for a chuckle. To a Younger Self trapped in some hellish moment of absolute mortification, it's no joke at all!

Being a fat kid at school is no picnic, but that level of humiliation might seem *vastly* preferable to the complex social nightmare of being "attractive." Putting on weight can be a more or less successful attempt to exit that arena, by becoming romantically invisible. Especially after a devastating rejection.

That Was Then, This is Now

So what's the big deal? Even if adolescence was horrible, an absolute nightmare, that was a long time ago. How could that be keeping you from losing weight today?

As adults those terrible experiences are just memories that we may hardly ever think about. In fact, we may have forgotten all about them. But remember, for our Younger Selves these are current events that never stop happening.

Why is that important? Because your decision to buckle down and lose some weight may actually trigger one or more of your Younger Selves, breaching that protective layer of dissociation. Their feelings can come flooding into your body now. What sort of feelings? There could be shame, disgust, anxiety or even terror. Given the awful experience they're having, it's going to be pretty bad.

This surge of negative emotions may or may not rise to the level of your conscious awareness, but it *will* likely have a powerful effect, overwhelming whatever motivation prompted you to make your decision. You may find yourself binge eating before you know what hit you.

Faulty Code

If you think of your brain as a computer, whatever decisions your Younger Self made in that moment of distress are like lines of code running in your subconscious operating system. Here are possible examples:

Being thin is dangerous
Losing weight is dangerous
Being attractive is dangerous
Feeling attractive is dangerous
Being safe is the top priority
Fat makes me invisible
Fat makes me safe

I can't trust myself (because I want to feel good)
It's not safe to feel good about my body
Feeling good draws attention
Feeling disgusted makes me safe
Shame makes me safe

If you adopted any of these beliefs as the result of unwanted sexual attention, they're likely to be strongly charged emotionally and actually given priority over health, fitness or aesthetic concerns. Your subconscious will do anything it can to keep you safe, even if it kills you!

Do You Have an On-Off Switch?

Years ago, I saw a documentary about Marilyn Monroe. A friend was describing a time they were out shopping in Manhattan, just walking down the busy sidewalks. Weirdly enough, nobody was noticing Marilyn at all.

This astonished the friend because Marilyn was at the peak of her fame. It was as though she was invisible. She finally mentioned it to Marilyn, who said "Hey, do you want to see something crazy?"

Without moving a muscle, just standing there looking her friend in the eyes, something about Marilyn changed. Suddenly everyone saw her and within moments she was mobbed by people clamoring for an autograph or photo. Their shopping trip was abruptly ended.

How did Marilyn do it? Clearly, she had some way of deliberately turning her visibility on or off. Might this be available to any of us? Something we could learn how to do? I honestly don't know, but it sure would be a *lot* more convenient than putting on weight.

It might be even more convenient to not be afraid anymore. To feel no shame, insecurity or the need to be invisible. The tapping script below may be helpful.

Tapping for Fear of Sexual Attention

Tapping on the karate chop point:

Even though the only way I can *possibly* be safe is to stay as heavy as possible, I still deeply love and completely accept myself.

And tapping through the points:

I want to lose weight
I need to lose weight
But there's no way in hell I'm ever going to let *that* happen
It's not safe
If I lose weight I'll be noticed
And it's not safe to be noticed
I can't handle it
And maybe bad things will happen
Maybe very bad things
If I let go of this weight I'll become more attractive

And part of me totally wants that
I forgive that part of me
She's forgotten what got attracted before
All of that creepy, gross attention
It was so scary
And so disgusting and horrible
I can never let that happen again
Being safe is the most important thing of all
And all of this fat makes me safe
I can't possibly give that up, that would be crazy

If I lose weight I'll get hit on
I'll stop being invisible
It will be exactly the same as before
Just as scary
Even though I'm older now
Even though I'm an adult
I'm still a child inside
I can't protect myself
I can't handle it
It's so incredibly scary
I'll just freeze up
I'll be defenseless
This fear of being noticed
Of being more attractive
Attractive to disgusting creeps
Attractive to monsters

Part of me wants to be sexy
And I forgive that part of me
But she must never get control
I should gain MORE weight
I should get more fat
What happened before will happen again
It's the only thing that can happen
The only thing that could ever happen
I can't even trust myself
I don't dare lose any weight
I need to be heavier

If I let anyone near me I'll be hurt
I'll be destroyed
I want to be loved so bad I can't trust myself
I'll let the wrong person in and they'll hurt me
I'll fall in love and betray myself
I have no way to protect myself
Except being fat
What happened before will happen again
Even though I'm not the same person I was
Even though I'm not a child
It feels like nothing has changed
This fear of being noticed
This fear of being hurt and used
This shame and disgust
This feeling of dread even thinking about it

I forgive myself for feeling powerless
I'm NOT who I was back then
I have learned a lot and I *do* have personal power
I CAN set healthy boundaries
I can tell people to fuck off
I know how to get help if I need it
I don't have to freeze up
I can actually fight back if I need to
And maybe I won't need to
Maybe I'm already safe
Whether I'm heavy or not
What if no one even wants to hurt me now?
What if I can protect myself, even if they do?
What if this extra fat isn't actually keeping me safe?

I can be cautious without being afraid
What happened before put me in shock
Maybe I've been in shock this whole time
The bad thing already happened
I choose to consider the idea that I'm actually safe now
That I don't have to be afraid anymore
That however much I weigh, it doesn't matter
I give myself permission to wake up from the shock

The shock of being violated
The shock that someone would do that
The shock that paralyzed me at the time
I give myself permission to come back to life
To reinhabit my body
I love myself for doing this tapping
I love myself for wanting to be free
Fearless and free

Younger-Self Tapping

On the karate chop point:

Even though you've been hurt and you're so freaked out
right now, you're not alone, I'm here to help you.

Tapping through the points:

What happened to you was so wrong
And so scary
And I think you may be in shock right now
But you're not alone
I'm here to help you
All of this fear
All of this shock
And you may be feeling so much shame
There's so much shame here
But it's not *your* shame
You've done nothing wrong at all
All of this shame is coming from the one who hurt you

This feeling of shock
This can't be happening
It's so wrong and bad
But *you're* not bad
This doesn't change who you are
You're a wonderful kid
And I want you to know this wasn't your fault
It didn't happen because you are bad
It happened because he's bad

All of this shame belongs to him, not you
And this is your body
It belongs to you
And he had no right to treat you like that

I'm so sorry this happened
That you weren't protected
And that you didn't know what to do
You didn't know how to make it stop
But I want you to know you deserve to be safe
You didn't deserve for this to happen
And I'm here to help you now
You're not alone

I don't want you to get stuck here
It's not your fault this happened
You deserve to feel safe again
You deserve to feel good about your own body
You don't need to be invisible now
You don't need to hide anymore
You aren't yucky
You aren't shameful
You are a wonderful kid worthy of love
It's okay to let this go now
I've got you

CHAPTER 9

Fear of Loss

Years ago I was trying to help a client stop smoking. As we tapped, he suddenly realized that if we were successful, he would lose his entire social life. This was a man with very few friends, or maybe no real friends at all. Smoke breaks at work were the *only* time he got to socialize with other human beings. The prospect of losing those connections was a terrifying show stopper.

So let me ask you something. If you were to attain and maintain your ideal weight, especially if it happened easily without a lot of struggle and bother, would your friends and family notice? If so, would they be happy for you?

Or not? Might you risk somehow offending them, hurting their feelings, or making them feel even worse about themselves? Maybe even inciting jealousy or envy?

Even if your friends *were* genuinely delighted in your weight loss success, might you be risking a loss of connection, with no more shared weight-loss obsession? A client once told me "Oh god, all of my friends are fat. That's pretty much all we talk about. That's our bond."

For some people, this fear of losing friends can be pretty intense. It can definitely be a Secret Reason for keeping weight on. This can be especially true if we have a Younger Self who was targeted, shunned or ostracized by false friends. Subconsciously, this is such a painful, devastating experience that it *must* be avoided at all costs. Staying heavy may seem like a small price to pay.

You might be thinking "With friends like that who needs enemies?" Fair to say, but you might have Younger Selves who don't know that yet, and *their* fear may be keeping you stuck.

All in the Family

This whole thing can get kicked up a notch when it's not just friends but family we're afraid of losing, or being attacked by. Mom, sisters, a close cousin. Do you have any family members you might lose if you attained your perfect weight?

Growing up, Sally's mom was loving but chronically busy and distracted. There never seemed to be time for doing anything special, no bedtime stories, no going shopping together or teaching Sally how to cook. Even with homework and school projects Sally was on her own. But there was one exception.

Mom was a hard-core dieter and when Sally was about 6 years old and maybe just a bit pudgy, mom began to take notice. This was a whole new world for Sally, mom fussing over how much she was eating, visits to the bathroom scale, and eventually getting scooped into the latest fad diet.

Finally, there was a way to connect with mom, to share something important to her, to have her ear and talk endlessly about their newly shared obsession. I should mention that mom was not overbearing or shaming. Her concern was motherly and felt absolutely wonderful to Sally.

Now 36 years later, the struggle to lose weight is *still* Sally's only real connection with mom. Their only way to be close. Can you imagine the potential bind here for

Sally? If she finally does succeed and slims down to her desired weight – and stays there with no real effort, what will mom think? How will mom feel?

Even if Sally is absolutely certain that her mom would be thrilled, that there would be *no* loss in their connection whatsoever, that they might grow even closer – her Younger Selves are likely to pitch a fit. Adult Sally's weight success would register as catastrophic for them, a return to the hell of emotional abandonment.

Do you see how this works? The Younger Selves are trapped in their own time and story. They don't really know about adult Sally, but become activated or triggered whenever she starts to slim down. That registers as a terrible risk of loss for them.

And they'll find a way to stop it. For them it's an urgent matter of self-protection. For Sally it will seem like absolute self-sabotage.

Living for Others

This *should* go without saying but I'll say it anyway: Anyone who cares for you should be delighted by your weight loss success. Rather than hurt or jealous, they should be inspired and perhaps keenly interested in how you pulled it off. If they can't manage that basic level of healthy relating, it's because something is wrong with them.

It's not your job to appease such people. You can't help them by playing small or staying heavy. No matter how much misery may love company, your weight loss success is actually a gift to those around you. It's an opportunity to be inspired and to celebrate with you. Whether they can receive that gift is not something you can control.

You have every right to live your highest and best, most authentic life. To be happy and successful. Deep down I'm sure you know this is true, but those freaked-out Younger Selves might have some serious fear of loss, or of being all alone in the world. If so, we can help them!

Whether it's valid or not, fear tends to grow in the dark. Bringing our fears up into the light while tapping tends to put them into perspective. Sometimes they simply dissolve. We may even laugh at the absurdity of our childish fears in the context of our adult life now. How could we have been so afraid of that monster under the bed?

Even if your fear of loss *is* grounded in reality – that is, you really might inspire hostility or actually lose someone, tapping may give you the clarity to make difficult choices. What price are you willing to pay to keep someone in your life? If a relationship is that unhealthy, what are you actually getting out it? What is it costing you and is it worth it?

One of the things I love about EFT is that graceful solutions may suddenly occur to us. They were there all along, but hidden by the fear that we've just tapped away.

Loss of Identity

For some people, the thought of starting over in a new town where no one knows them is *very* appealing. The freedom to reinvent themselves, start from scratch, build a whole new life? How intoxicating! How many movies feature this plot line? There must be dozens and dozens.

On the other hand, I've known folks who would consider that a terrifying scenario. The familiar regard of the people they know, or of the people who at least recognize them, provides a sort of web that holds their sense of identity

The thought of losing that web isn't exciting; it's scary! Even if they're generally looked down upon, at least they're known. To some people who identify strongly with their bodies, making a significant change can feel as terrifying as moving to a new town. They're afraid that if they change too much, no one will recognize them. Without that recognition they fear that "I won't know who I am anymore."

Could this fear of losing your identity be a Secret Reason for you? If you're wanting significant weight loss, success would mean that you'd look physically different, right? In a good way, of course, but still quite different. You might also feel better about yourself. Maybe a lot better – more capable, disciplined and competent. A winner at losing! Losing weight, that is.

None of that should be a problem, should it? It's all really good stuff. Unless it taps into some sort of identity fear. We've all heard stories about people winning gazillions of dollars in the lottery, only to lose it all within a few years. Their sudden shift in identify must have triggered a compulsion to get rid of their riches.

Let's not let anything like that happen to you! Just a bit of tapping may turn anxiety into excitement. Let's welcome the loss of the old as simply making space for the new. I'd love to help you welcome your new improved identity as a wonderful upgrade.

Tapping for Fear of Loss of Friends*

*Or substitute whomever you might fear to lose.

Tapping on the karate chop point:

Even though I'm stuck – if I lose weight, I'll lose my friends and I can't let that happen – I still deeply love and completely accept myself.

Tapping through the points:

If I actually lose all this weight and keep it off
I'm totally going to lose my friends
All of my friends are fat
All of them struggle
It's the one thing we all have in common
They hate being fat
They hate themselves for being fat
But if I slim down they'll hate me
If I look good, that will make them feel worse about
themselves
If I slim down it'll be like slapping them in the face
They'll hate the sight of me
They'll hate being around me
I'll be making them look bad

Even if they don't really hate me
I know they'll be uncomfortable
They won't mean to, but how can they not feel bad about
it?
How can they not feel bad seeing me slim?
What if they secretly resent me?
Or what if it's *not* that secret?
If I don't stay fat I'm taking a terrible risk
I might lose all my friends and then I'll be alone
It's not easy making new friends
It's really hard!
They're the only friends I have
The only friends I'll ever have

How can I risk being totally alone forever?
Being shunned by the only ones who know me?
I can't bear the idea of being alone
Who will I hang out with?
Who even *cares* about me?
What the hell am I thinking, wanting to lose weight?
What a terrible idea!

I know if any of my friends lost weight
I'd totally resent them for it

There's no way I'd be happy for them
I'd be angry and hurt
How dare she make me look bad?
How could she *do* that to me?
There's no way I could be happy for my friend
I'd be bitter
I'd take it personally
I'd totally HATE her for losing all that weight!

Okay, actually, none of that is true
I wouldn't feel any of those things
Or at least I wouldn't *want* to
I'd be ashamed to hate my friend for losing weight
For being happier
And maybe I'd want to know how she did it
What finally worked for her?
What did the trick?
Why do I think my friends would hate *me* for losing
weight?
Why wouldn't they want to know how I did it?
Why wouldn't they be inspired?
What if they were actually happy for me?

I guess if they weren't happy for me
If they really were jealous or bitter
If they'd rather I stayed fat
I guess they wouldn't actually *be* friends
With friends like that, who needs enemies?

But I can't risk it!
What if they *are* mean and jealous?
What if they *do* abandon or shun me?
What if my worst fears are grounded?
What if my friends really are awful people?
If that were true, what am I actually getting out of our
friendship?
I guess if they're really *that* bad
Maybe I would be better off alone

But that's scary!
It really is hard to make new friends
At least it always has been
But what if I change so much for the better
That it actually gets easier and easier?
As my self-esteem gets better and better
Of course people will want to know me

I've been so afraid of being abandoned by my friends
What if I've misjudged them?
What if they're happy and inspired?
What if *my* losing weight helps them?
I've been too afraid to test the waters
To take the risk
And I forgive myself for that
But even if they dump me in an ugly way
I'll still be okay
And if that happened, I really would be better off without them
But maybe I wouldn't be alone very long anyway
With or without my old friends, I want to be happier
I want to be healthier
And I love myself for letting go of all this emotional weight

Tapping for Fear of Loss of Identity

Tapping on the karate chop point:

Even though if I lose weight I won't know who I am anymore, I give myself permission to find out.

Tapping through the points:

I'm just fat
That's all I am
That's all I ever think about
How fat I am
What I want to eat and how I shouldn't eat it
I'm so used to feeling bad about myself

About my body
I wouldn't know who I am if all of that drops away
I guess I'd be nobody
And being a fat body is better than a no-body!
I'm so afraid there's nothing else to me
Nothing else I'm even interested in
What would I do with my time?
What would I even think about?
What would I do if I wasn't so miserable and obsessed all
the time?

Maybe I'd like to find out
What would life be like if I were happier
Freer
If I had more time and energy
I *do* have interests
There's so much else I could be doing
Learning
Experiencing
My life has been so constrained
I've been so caught up in this weight issue
What if there's a whole world to explore?

I've been scared of that world
But why?
What if I find out who I really am
And actually *love* that new me?
I'm totally sick of the old me
So obsessed with weight and fat and food
I give myself permission to find out what else is out there
What else life has to offer me
I guess if I get to my ideal weight and hate it
I can always gain it all back
If I really want to
Maybe it really *is* safe to lose my old identity
And find a new one
I give myself permission to be brave
To be curious
To maybe even enjoy my new life

CHAPTER 10

Rebellion

Clara and I seemed to be making great progress, tapping on her weight-loss issue and feelings of self-loathing. She was yawning a lot, and with tapping that means the body is dumping massive amounts of stress. I was secretly patting myself on the back, when she let out a loud and angry exclamation: "I'll be damned if I let her win!"

I think Clara was just as surprised as I was, hearing these words come out of her mouth. But there was no mystery at all about who she wouldn't let win.

Clara's mom was a full-on narcissist. By that I mean she was unable to see her daughter as a real person, with her own needs, ideas and purpose. Rather, she was intent on *using* Clara to make herself look like the perfect mother.

That meant Clara, from a very young age, had to look and behave like a perfect little doll. Or else.

Unfortunately, many parents are more intent on controlling their children than helping them grow into successful, independent adults. Some might use harsh words and criticism. Others become cold and distant, invoking fears of abandonment. And of course, some use rage and beatings to dominate their children.

Clara's mother used all of the above, and in an unpredictable way that made it even worse.

So, from the time she was an infant, Clara had lived in a state of uncertainty and actual terror. There was no "terrible twos" phase for her. No saying "NO!" to mom. No teenage rebellion. Because of this, Clara's ability to set healthy boundaries with anyone was rather stunted. And just under the surface there was a lot of rage.

Despite cutting off all contact years earlier, it became clear she was still locked in a bitter power struggle with her mom. Or rather her Younger Selves were.

Every time Clara decided to lose weight, the specter of her mother's obsessive and overbearing demands was retriggered. Her Younger Selves' seething hatred of mom would be activated, and their long-thwarted rebellion transferred onto Clara!

She grimly described it as almost magical. Just the *thought* of dieting seemed to increase her weight. She didn't even need to eat anything!

I know that may sound crazy but I've actually heard the same story from other clients. They've been eating five sunflower seeds and half a stick of celery a day, yet they still gained 3 pounds. Okay, maybe they're exaggerating, but I pretty much believe them. The subconscious mind is incredibly powerful.

I've also come to appreciate what's at stake in this sort of power-struggle. It feels very much like a fight for survival. The survival of our Self as an individual. Giving in can feel like being extinguished as a person, as a real and separate individual.

In extreme cases like Clara's, it's worse than feeling like a humiliated slave. It's a kind of attempted soul murder. So yes, the stakes were high indeed.

Clearly her mother was off the deep end, but does any of this sound familiar to you? If not, that's great! You can pretty much skim through the rest of this chapter.

But if you *did* grow up with a controlling, domineering or overbearing parent, could it be that your own attempt to lose weight feels like losing a power struggle? Like giving in? Knuckling under? Hopefully your own parent wasn't *such* a nightmare as Clara's, but might you be inciting a rebellion simply by making healthy, adult decisions?

This past year, two different clients introduced me to an even deeper level of this control dynamic. After a good deal of tapping, they became aware of the odd sensation that their own body didn't really belong to them, and never had. For both clients this came as a sudden realization. They'd been living as though their own body was actually their parent's property, not their own!

That's a pretty spooky realization. In one case, my client had been compulsively negligent of her physical welfare. This had been going on for decades. With this new awareness, she likened it to borrowing a car from someone you absolutely hate and then returning it dirty and scratched up. Her overeating went beyond rebellion into actual revenge!

A less extreme way this might show up is when you eat something naughty. There might be a little extra pleasure or satisfaction in breaking the rules, in getting away with something, while eating that piece of chocolate. Shooting yourself in the foot (as far as losing weight goes) may be a small price to pay for the sake of that little thrill of "victory."

Your Attitude Can Be Healing

Growing up with a harsh or controlling parent, it's almost impossible not to soak up their negative attitude toward yourself. Whenever a Younger Self grabs the wheel, so to speak, and you end up "misbehaving" with food, how do you regard yourself? Do you automatically adopt your parents' harsh regard and manner toward yourself?

If so, the realization that you're acting *just like them* can be very unpleasant! Ugh!

But this is an important thing to get a handle on, because acting like your parents makes it *much* easier to inadvertently trigger your Younger Selves. They'll confuse you with mom or dad, and here comes the rebellion!

Another serious problem is this: the more we reject our own Younger Selves (the part of us that misbehaves), the more we condemn them, push them away and try to create distance, the more *autonomous* they become. This shows up as out-of-control compulsive behavior – not good!

Ideally, we'd like to have some influence with our Younger Selves. To help them get with the program, to join the team. Imagine actually getting their *help* instead of resistance or sabotage. Regarding them with shame, anger or rejection makes such an alliance pretty much impossible.

If you are a parent yourself, hopefully you've found it natural to express kindness and affection toward your own children. But you also know this can be extremely difficult when they are misbehaving. When working with your Younger Selves, the ability to express genuine care in the face of their rebellion is immensely helpful.

The fact is, their urge for rebellion against a domineering parent is actually healthy, maybe even life-saving. We can validate their feelings, while helping them distinguish between their parent and you.

If you've never experienced that kind of healthy unconditional positive regard that parents are *supposed* to have toward their children, that's okay. It's a learnable (and life-changing) skillset and mindset.

When rebellion is the Secret Reason for keeping the weight on, a kind, loving, and respectful attitude toward ourself and our Younger Selves is absolutely essential. Especially when we've been "misbehaving"!

Tapping for Rebellion

Tapping on the karate chop point:

Even though I'll never lose weight because I'll be damned if I let her win, I still deeply love and completely accept myself.

Tapping through the points

If I lose weight she wins
That's my story and I'm sticking to it
I never got to just be a kid
I never got to eat what I wanted
I was forced to be her little doll
And I'll never get over it
Never in a million years
What she did to me was a crime
She stole my childhood from me
And for what?
To try and make herself look good?
She can go to hell!

I'll never give her the satisfaction
I'll never give in
She controlled me and still would if I let her
Fuck you mom!
Fuck you and your obsession with MY body
It's *my* body, not yours
You had no right to control me that way
And now I can't control myself

I can't control my eating
And it's your goddamned fault!

Dieting feels like giving in to her
Like being under her thumb again
Like letting her win and I won't do it
I'm going to *gain* weight just to spite her
I'll do whatever it takes to embarrass her
To show the world she has no control over me
To prove that *I'm* the one calling the shots

Except I really *do* want to lose weight
I really do want to slim down
I have my own reasons
Legitimate reasons
But it's just not worth it
I can't let her win
Even though I've cut her out of my life
She's living rent-free in my head
Every time I try to control my own diet
It's like giving in to her demands
I want her out of my head

I forgive myself for still being locked in this battle
This endless conflict with her
It's not even her, really
It's my awful memory of her
And what she did to me
If I really want to win, I need to forget her
To stop being so angry

I have every *right* to be angry
I have every right to feel *rage* at what she did to me
And I have every right to let it go
It's not costing her anything
But it's costing me dearly
It's costing me my freedom to have what I want

I want to be free to know what *I* want
To make my own choices

Not out of rebellion
Not in opposition
That's just me still being connected to her
I choose to *disconnect* as best I can
If this anger is keeping me connected
I choose to let it go
To release this totally justified anger
I want to get to a peaceful place inside
A place where I'm free to make my own choices
The freedom I never had as a child

And even though my mom demanded I be skinny
I choose to lose weight for my own reasons
For my own happiness
And that's the real winning
That's the best revenge – being happy
Being true to myself
I have every right to hold on to this anger
But I'd like to forget she even exists
To never think of her
For days or weeks or months at a time
To enjoy my own body
Enjoy the freedom to be my own person
To eat or not eat whatever I want
However much I want
With no mom in the equation

I want all of my Younger Selves to know
I am NOT mom
Controlling my diet is NOT giving in
Losing weight is NOT letting her win
Refraining from sweets is NOT losing
Being in charge of myself is winning
Losing weight is winning
Being happy is winning

Younger-Self Tapping for Rebellion

Tapping on the karate chop point:

Even though you're so angry about being controlled, you are not alone, I'm here to help you.

Tapping through the points:

You have every right to be angry
The way she treats you is not okay, it's wrong
She never lets you do what you want
She never lets you be who you want to be
She doesn't even care what you want
It's her way or else
She's so scary and so mean
And you have every right to be angry
You have every right to stamp your foot and scream NO!

You're a real person with your own needs
But she treats you like her puppet
You're just here to make *her* look good
And that's not how a real mom is supposed to act
She doesn't care about what *you* need
She only wants to control you
And I know how scary it is to say no
It's so scary to go against her
There's hell to pay if you piss her off
It's not safe to make her mad at you
Or at least it doesn't feel safe

I'm you from the future
And I want you to know it won't always be this way
You are going to grow up and leave home
You won't have to live with her forever
You won't have to listen to her
Or do what she says
You're going to have your own life
And do what YOU want to do
I promise

But it's so important to start letting go
To let go of caring so much about her
I don't want you to make the same mistake I did

I left home but carried her with me in my head
I couldn't stop thinking about her
And feeling really mad
You have every *right* to be mad at her
But it keeps you connected to her all the time
It means you're always thinking about her
And I want you to have your own thoughts about your
own life

Even though she has so much power over you right now
It's *your* life, not hers
You have your own thoughts
Your own feelings
Your own ideas
Your own inner life
You're going to grow up and have your own life

Maybe it's good to stay out of trouble
You can't really ignore her yet
She's still too scary
She can still mess with you
But you can learn to not care so much
To not take it personally
There's just something *wrong* with her
She's kind of broken in a way
And it's not your job to fix her
It's not your job to try and get her to love you
To respect you
To treat you nice
She's messed up and just can't do it

But other people can
Other people will love you and see who you really are
You're a wonderful kid
You have every right to be angry
And you have every right to start letting it go
If it keeps you tied to her, it's okay to stop caring so much
You can feel good about who you are without any help
from her

You're a wonderful kid and you have every right to be
happy

I know it's almost impossible right now
But if you can keep from taking mom with you
In your own head
You might just have a better life than I've had
I want to lose weight, to get skinnier
But I just get so mad at how she controlled me
It feels like she's winning
I want better for you
You get to decide what you want
Even if it's what she wanted too
You have your own reasons that have nothing to do with
her

CHAPTER 11

Deprivation

O f all of the Secret Reasons, deprivation may be the most understandable. If you've ever endured a time when food was scarce, experienced serious physical hunger, or a time in your past when you were desperate for anything sweet or yummy, then you know how intense it can be. And you likely have a very hungry Younger Self stuck there.

We've talked about how a Younger Self's feelings of anxiety, shame, anger, fear or whatever, can come flooding into your body now, essentially hijacking your present experience. But what about feelings of physical hunger? Are there times you might be feeling a Younger Self's intense hunger as if it were your own?

If that's actually possible, do you think that you eating something *now* would somehow help your Younger Self back in her time? I'm pretty sure the answer is no.

If your urge to binge is coming from the hunger of a Younger Self, no matter how much you eat *she* won't be satisfied. Rather, the binge likely ends when our feeling sick enough now overrides the feelings of hunger coming from the past. In other words, maybe we binge until we are in more distress than our Younger Self.

Even if we're not experiencing a Younger Self's feelings of physical hunger, our desire to eat less or cut down on sugar might trigger their deprivation trauma, causing their feelings of *emotional* distress to flood into us. This can be a strong subconscious pushback against our healthy adult choices.

In my work I've run into a number of different deprivation scenarios, each one with its own peculiar spin. In no particular order, here are some of the situations I've helped clients deal with.

Actual Hunger

Mary grew up in a South American country with two older sisters and a mom with mental health issues. When Mary was turning 7, dad totally abandoned the family and left them penniless. Mom struggled to manage but there was never enough to eat and for several years Mary endured actual hunger on a daily basis.

Mom did have family nearby but they looked down their noses at her and her three unkempt children. Help was sporadic and always doled out with a heavy dose of shaming.

Speaking of shame, when Mary was finally able to go to school, she was chronically hungry. One day she saw a crust of bread on the playground and grabbed it without even thinking, stuffing it into her mouth. Some of the other kids witnessed this, which did *not* help Mary's social standing!

Fast forward 20 years; Mary is beautiful, successful and *hates* herself for being fat. Locked in an endless struggle to lose weight, she's just so tired of the obsession and feeling miserable. We started off by tapping on her intense self-loathing (see chapter 6) and I'm not sure I've ever seen anyone let it go so fast.

This was great, since we had quite a few Younger Selves who really needed help. As we got them sorted out, one by one, Mary's Secret Reason around deprivation just melted away. This was a story with a happy ending.

The Mad Scramble

Margie had enough will power to refrain from buying chocolate and bringing it home, but if anyone brought some to work or a party, watch out! In fact, Margie had embarrassed herself more than once, compulsively gobbling down sweets in a social setting. She clearly had a Younger Self "grabbing the wheel."

Growing up with lots of siblings in a rather poor family, treats were few and far between. When something yummy did show up, there was no doling it out. Nothing fair about it. "The Fast and the Full, the Slow and the Hungry" seemed to be their family motto. As one of the younger kids, Margie found it hard to ever get her share (or any at all) in the mad scramble. This drama was repeated *many* times over the course of her childhood.

Barely scratching the surface of these memories brought up all kinds of hard feelings, which we were able to tap away in short order. Margie's cravings for chocolate and sweets were released along with her old trapped emotions of scarcity, desperation and resentment. Done and dusted.

The Blitz

Janet was born in London, near the end of WWII. Dad was away fighting in the war, leaving his pregnant wife to manage with two young children amid the shambles of the bombing. Food was scarce and for a time Janet's mother struggled to feed her family. Janet was born into an environment of terrible ongoing distress.

Fortunately, everything turned out all right for Janet and her family. The war ended, Dad came home, and they muddled through the post-war scarcities. But while Janet was in the womb, she was intimately sharing her mother's emotional experience of the war. All of Mom's fear and insecurity over not having enough food was carried in her blood stream, coming right into Janet's body through the umbilical cord and recorded in every cell.

From the very beginning of her life, Janet's tiny body was being programmed to hold onto every possible scrap of energy, storing it as fat. Her subconscious set-point for weight was recalibrated before she was even born!

This is actually a well-known phenomenon after disasters of mass starvation, such as the Dutch *Hongerwinter* during WWII and the Great Chinese Famine, when millions starved to death due to Mao's disastrous agricultural policies. Compared to siblings conceived before or after a famine, children conceived *during* the famine were typically born small and underweight, and at increased risk for obesity if they survived.

A long and seemingly impossible struggle to lose weight somehow led Janet to me. She was beyond frustrated. Nothing ever seemed to work in the slightest. And to be honest, this was a tough job even for EFT tapping! We had to reach the Younger Self all the way back in the womb, releasing the fear and distress she'd picked up from mom.

This was not a quick fix. It took persistence, but ultimately, we were successful.

Unfortunate Punishment

Compared to war and famine, being sent to bed without any supper might seem like no big deal. Weirdly though, the effect on a young child can be nearly as severe. Since our parents are the people *most* in charge of our wellbeing, tying punishment for unacceptable behavior to issues of basic survival is actually kind of extreme.

It's not just the deprivation of food; it's also the deprivation of love and respect.

Of course, missing out on dinner isn't actually life-threatening, but try telling that to a 3- or 4-year-old. Even a 6-year-old. Their fear might surprise you. Lying in bed, trying to fall asleep with a growling empty belly is no joke. I hope this never happened to you as a child, but if it did, this could definitely be a Secret Reason why you can't lose weight.

As an adult, your decision to eat less, cut out meals or lay off the sweets may cast *you* in the role of the punishing parent, inciting rebellion or actual fear in your Younger Self. Intermittent fasting might make a lot of sense on the biological level, but not if it's causing an emotional shit show behind the scenes.

Withholding dessert or sweets as punishment has got to be less destructive than sending a child to bed hungry, but how many of us decide to forego the *crème brûlée* only to suffer blowback from a Younger Self who confuses us with their mean, unloving parent?

Milk of Human Kindness

Several times now, I've seen at least part of a client's weight problem go back to breastfeeding issues in infancy. In one case, his mother was unable to produce enough milk so my client was chronically hungry as a baby. This installed a scarcity program, telling his body to hold on to extra calories for dear life.

Another woman I worked with experienced her mother's milk as sour and unpalatable. This seemed to set her up for an endless quest for sweetness, especially through food and drink.

If you've heard stories of problems with breastfeeding or formula in your own infancy, it might be helpful directing the words of your tapping toward that little baby, possibly helping her feel safer and more content.

Love Contaminated with Fear

Alan had a great dad, who clearly loved him very much. The problem we worked on is that, as a boy, his dad would urge Alan to keep eating until he was too full. This happened pretty much on a nightly basis.

There was no element of punishment. No "You can't leave the table until you've cleaned your plate" kind of harshness. Rather, his dad was expressing some sort of deep concern for Alan's welfare. Alan could feel this, could see it in his father's eyes. It was an expression of love, but love contaminated with fear.

His father's strange anxiety and insistence to keep eating overrode Alan's own internal sense of being full, setting him up for a lifetime of overeating he was now struggling to overcome.

It turned out that Alan's dad was a young boy when the Great Depression hit. In the first months of the crisis, the whole community was truly frightened – his parents, the neighbors, the teachers at school. No one knew how long it would last or whether there would be enough food to survive.

As it turned out, dad's family and his local community weathered the hard times better than most and no one ended up going hungry. By the time the atmosphere of distress had mellowed though, the damage was done for Alan's dad. He'd picked up a fear of food scarcity that never left him. A fear he conveyed to his son nightly by urging him to "eat up."

I've noticed whenever the love of a parent is contaminated by fear, the fear tends to get deep into us. We have no resistance to it.

In helping Alan, we ended up doing a sort of generational healing for his father's Younger Self. This is an advanced level of EFT work beyond the scope of this book and best done with a trained practitioner. Not because it's risky or dangerous *per se*, but it does tend to be rather complex.

That said, simply tapping on every aspect of the situation that holds an emotional charge could definitely help and possibly "do the trick."

Tapping for Deprivation

Here is a tapping script to help take the charge off of possible deprivation issues. If any particular lines don't apply to your history, no worries. Saying them out loud won't hurt you in any way. Or feel free to skip whatever doesn't fit.

Tapping on the karate chop point:

Even if I have some deep-rooted fear of deprivation running in my body or subconscious mind, right now I'm in no danger of going hungry, and I deeply love and completely accept myself.

Tapping through the points:

There's no way I can lose weight
No matter how much I want to slim down
I need every scrap of energy I can get
Every scrap of energy stored as fat in my body
Or at least that seems to be what's happening
It's not safe to be hungry
It's not safe to deny myself any type of food
Even if it's junk food
Even if it's unhealthy for me
I need every calorie I can get
Stored as fat
Or else

This fear
This fear of starvation
This fear of *death* from starvation
This old, old fear that has *no* basis in reality now
My poor body is living in the past
When there really was a time of fear
A time when I really *was* hungry
When I may have actually thought I would die!

The good news is it never happened
I made it through just fine
And I'm in no danger of starving now
Not even of going hungry
But the fear!
The fear is there
Right under the surface
This fear of going hungry
This fear of missing a meal
Of not cleaning my plate
Of not getting enough

I need to eat until I'm stuffed
The food may run out at any time
There's not enough to go around
What if I can't find enough to eat?
What if I starve to death?
All of this fear
This fear of hunger
This fear of losing weight

Extra fat makes my body feel safer
It feels like safety
I want my body to know we're just as safe without it
Maybe even safer
All of this fear
This fear of being thin
This fear of losing weight
This fear of going hungry
This fear of not being full

I forgive myself for any and all fear still running in my
system

I *will* die one day
Or at least my body will
But probably not for a very long time
And probably not from starvation
I will always have enough to eat
I will always be safe from hunger
And I want to live without this fear
Without this feeling of emergency

I give my body permission to feel hunger without fear
To feel my stomach emptying out with no panic
To actually feel full when I've eaten *just* enough
I give my body permission to relax fully and completely
I give my body permission to feel safe

All this fear
This fear of being hungry
This fear of losing weight
This fear of being skinny
This fear of having a thin body
This fear of losing too much fat
Of losing *any* fat
This fear of going without sweets
This fear of going without an extra helping
This fear of *not* cleaning my plate
This fear there won't be enough
All this fear around starvation
Of lack
Of hunger
Of dying

I forgive myself for having these fears
I love myself for wanting to finally feel safe in this body
I love my body for wanting to keep me safe
I love myself for knowing that I *am* safe

Tapping for a Younger Self's Fear of Hunger

Tapping on the karate chop point:

Even though you're so hungry right now, you're going to be okay and I'm here to help you.

Tapping through the points:

It must feel so bad being hungry
I bet you feel scared
It's okay, you're going to make it through this
You're going to be okay
I promise
I'm *you* from the future and I'm still here
I'm living proof that you're not going to die of hunger
Even if it's uncomfortable
Even if it's scary
It's okay to relax
I know it feels bad
But you don't have to be scared

It's not your fault this is happening to you
It's not because you are bad
It's not because you deserve it
You're a wonderful kid
You deserve to be full and safe and happy
Whatever is happening right now isn't going to last
Things will get back to normal
You're going to be okay again

There's going to be enough to eat
Maybe not right now
But soon enough
I know it feels bad
You have every right to be upset
But I don't want you to be scared
I promise you aren't going to die from this

If someone is keeping you from eating
That's not okay
They shouldn't be doing that
It's stupid and really mean
But it's not your fault
You don't deserve it

All of this fear
Your stomach may be growling
It may feel *so* empty
But you're still totally safe
Even if it doesn't feel very nice
I want you to know you're not alone
I felt your fear and have come back to help you
I promise you'll be okay
It's okay to ignore your empty stomach
It's okay to think about other things
It's okay to feel safe now
You're going to be okay
I promise

Obsessive Thinking

How much "mental real estate" does your weight issue take up? I've had clients tell me that obsessive thinking was actually the worst part of their whole weight loss problem.

They were so consumed with obsessive thoughts about what to eat, what not to eat, what they could or couldn't "get away with," who might be judging them, needing to exercise, hating to exercise, clothing issues, and on and on, that they could hardly stand it.

If that sounds familiar, here's another question: If you *weren't* spending so much time and mental energy obsessing on your weight issue, what might you be thinking about instead? And what might you be doing?

If we're successful in helping you tap away your Secret Reasons and you're finally able to attain and maintain your ideal weight, effortlessly with no more exhausting obsession...a whole lot of mental space may open up for you.

But nature abhors a vacuum, right? So, what might take the place of all your weight angst?

Dangerous Aspirations

Is there some project, challenge or achievement you've always dreamed of tackling? Going back to school, learning to play the guitar, trying for that big promotion, taking French lessons, signing up for an improv class?

If there *is* something compelling that you'd love to do, does the thought of pursuing it bring up some kind of fear? Maybe fear of failure, disappointment or rejection? Is it possible that your obsessive thinking about weight might be protecting you from 'going for it'?

The possibility of failure can be uncomfortable, but when it feels *inevitable,* that's a real problem. And it just might seem inevitable if you're burdened with low self-esteem and a distorted sense of your own capabilities. When it comes to some important dream that's truly dear to our heart, our "inevitable" failure would be devastating, right?

Instead of inspiration, our beloved goal or dream might bring us dread. We might even experience it as a kind of burden.

Here then is a potential Secret Reason for keeping your weight on. Obsessive thinking may be protecting you from your own seemingly "dangerous" aspirations.

Just in case this might be true, let me suggest taking a few minutes to jot down any "dangerous" goals, achievements, projects or desires you might have on the back burner. There may even be a list of them. Pinpointing these will be helpful in the tapping we'll be doing.

Better the Devil You Know

Aside from the painful fear of failure, obsessing over weight issues might be fending off those loss-of-identity fears we looked at in Chapter 9: "If I stop obsessing about this weight problem, who will I be? I won't know who I am anymore!"

"Who will I be?" could actually be an exciting question to ask, full of wonderful possibilities. Unless perhaps you have a Younger Self who decided she's bad, unlovable, incapable or worthless. Then it might be a very scary question indeed.

Obsessing about weight sucks, but at least it's familiar territory. Better the devil you know, right?

If you're reading this book, *I* believe you are destined for greater things than struggling to lose weight. I'm certain of it. How do we restore your faith in your own potential? Stay with me and we'll try some tapping at the end of this chapter.

That Voice in Your Head

If you suffer from obsessive thinking about your weight issue, does that include having a critical voice in your head that offers a running commentary on your life? If not, halleluiah! You can just skim through this section. But if you *do* have a voice that plagues you, read on.

Whether it's about weight or any other issue, many people have a critical voice in their head offering up a corrosive and unpleasant narration of everything they do, basically undermining and tarnishing their experience of life. As far as I can make out, that voice is *never* helpful. To the contrary, it seems dedicated to tearing us down.

Here's another question: If you do have a voice like that, does it say "I" or does it say "You"? For example, say you're eyeing a piece of chocolate; would the voice say something like: "Mmmm, that looks so good, but I really shouldn't eat that." Or would it be more like: "OMG, are you serious? You are *such* a pig!"? You see the difference, right?

Here's the thing, we never refer to ourselves as "You." Try it and I guarantee it'll sound totally crazy. So if the voice in your head is saying "You" instead of "I," that means it's *not your voice.*

Which begs two questions. 1) If it's not *your* voice, whose voice is it?

I'm going to go out on a limb here and suggest it's probably either mom or dad. I've noticed that's almost always the case. What do you think?

Question 2) How did this voice get into your head? I've got some ideas, but first of all, let me assure you that whoever the voice sounds like, it's not really them. Dad, for example, is not down in his basement (or beyond the grave) broadcasting into your head with a tiny transmitter. But if it really seems like his voice, how did it get there?

Here's what I think happens. As children we hate getting in trouble. It's scary at best, but in some families it might actually be dangerous. To avoid this terrible fate, many clever children begin to *anticipate* what our mom or dad might say about whatever potential mischief they may be considering.

Over time, this "What would dad say?" protection can become habitual and take on a life of its own. We end up internalizing a hyper-critical version of one or both of our parents, and we do this out of anxiety or even fear. Initially it's there to help keep us safe, so we may end up giving that voice a lot of authority.

As adults, this voice is *not* very helpful in keeping us out of trouble. We'll eat the chocolate anyway and then let the voice beat us up for it. Rather than helping us stay out of trouble, the voice itself becomes the punisher and an ongoing source of low self-esteem. Which in turn drives overeating.

The voice may have actually worked somewhat in childhood, but I promise you'll be much better off without it. Let's see if we can tap it away, or at least turn its volume way, way down.

Tapping for Obsessive Thinking and the Critical Voice

Tapping on the karate chop point:

Even though I can't stop thinking about losing weight, and every time I blow it I get so down on myself, I choose to forgive myself for that. I choose to love and accept myself anyway, as best I can.

Tapping through the points:

I'm *so* obsessed with losing weight
With what I want to eat
And how I shouldn't eat it
And what I should eat instead
And how my clothes are fitting
And how much weight I just put on
And how ugly I look
And how everyone must judge me
I can hardly stand it
I can't stand these thoughts in my own head
It's too much
There's not enough room for anything else!

This endless stream of unpleasant thoughts
It's so depressing
There's no joy in any of it
But I can't help it
It's not something I'm doing on purpose
It's just happening to me

I'm so sick of thinking about weight and fat and food
And I'm sick of all the bad feelings that go with those
thoughts

I'm a failure
I'm unacceptable
I'm too fat
I should try harder
I have no will power
I want to eat something sweet and that's wrong
My clothes don't fit
What are people going to think when they see me?
I'm such a loser
All of these ugly unhelpful thoughts in my head

And that horrible, critical voice
Just in case I forget, it's always there to remind me
I have no right to feel good
I can't forget for a moment
This weight struggle is the *only* thing that matters
I have no right to forget it
And everything I do is always wrong
Everything I want to eat is wrong
I mustn't forget how freaking important it is to lose
weight
And what a failure I am

I hate that voice in my head
I just want peace
I just want to live in the moment
I want to stop hearing that stupid voice

What if I could just turn it off?
Or turn the volume down?
What if I didn't even *care* what it said?
What if I actually found the voice funny?
OMG, what's it saying now? That's hilarious!

What if I could just roll my eyes when it's ragging on me?
Or roll my third eye
What if I found the voice ridiculous?
What if it became impossible to take it seriously?
Impossible to take any of what it's saying personally

I forgive myself for installing this voice
I don't remember doing it, but I must have
Maybe I needed it to stay out of trouble
But I don't need it anymore
I don't have to listen
It's not helping me in any way
It's just a big drag
And I don't have to give it my attention anymore

If I stop hearing it though,
What will it be like in my head?
What will I hear if the voice is really gone?
OMG, maybe I'll get to hear my *own* thoughts
Maybe I'll find out who I really am
Without all of this struggle

Is that scary?
I don't think so
I don't know what I'll do with my life
Once this weight drama is over
But I want to find out
I choose to trust myself
I choose to trust my own voice, my own thoughts
My own feelings
What am I *really* here to do?
I want to know
And I choose to have faith in myself

Younger-Self Tapping for Getting in Trouble

Tapping on the karate chop point:

Even though it's scary getting in trouble, you're still a good kid and you're going to be okay, I promise.

Tapping through the points:

Sometimes mom/dad gets really angry
It's so scary
Maybe it seems like they don't even love you
Or that they want to *hurt* you
And that they think you're bad
That you're a bad kid because you did something wrong
Or something dumb
Or something careless

But even if they get really mad at you
Even if they think you really *are* bad
You're NOT a bad kid
You're a great kid and they're lucky to have you
Even if they forget that sometimes, it's still true

Everyone makes mistakes
They made mistakes too, when they were little
I bet they got in trouble and felt bad
And now they're acting just like *their* mom or dad
Now they get to be the powerful one
They probably don't know it
But maybe they're treating you the same way they got treated
And none of *that* is your fault

All kids make mistakes
Grown-ups make mistakes too
Sometimes we make big mistakes and break stuff
Or hurt someone
As long as you're not doing it on purpose
You get to make mistakes sometimes
It should be okay with mom/dad
But maybe they're too messed up

Maybe it reminds them of when *they* were little
And they just can't help it; they get mean

I just want you to know it won't always be this way
You're a great kid and have every right to feel good about
who you are
You don't have to be perfect to be loved
You get to make mistakes just like everyone else
You don't have to feel bad about who you are
You don't have to take it personally when mom/dad gets
mean
They're kind of broken, but it's not your job to fix them
It's not your job to stay out of trouble or else
It's your job to be *you*, and to be as happy as you can be

I promise they're not going to kill you!
I'm you from the future and I promise you'll get through
this
You're going to be okay
You don't have to worry so much
In fact, you don't really need to worry at all
Mom and dad are so lucky to have a kid like you

CHAPTER 13

Fear of Dating and Relationships

If you're single (and don't want to be) have you ever thought to yourself: "I'm not going to start dating again until I lose this weight"? Isn't that just another way of saying "I'm never going to lose this weight"?

I don't think I've ever met anyone who liked dating. For most of us it's uncomfortable at best. A potentially expensive, time consuming, awkward ordeal we'd definitely avoid if it wasn't the main gateway to relationship.

Using fat as an excuse to avoid the horrors of dating, or the potentially scarier prospect of getting into an actual relationship, may be one of the sneakier Secret Reasons. Sneaky because even if we really *are* lonely, even just one terrible experience can keep us stuck.

Let's take a look at some of the perils of dating and possible reasons for anti-dating emotional intensity.

What's Wrong with Dating?

Dating gives us an opportunity to explore the fine line between putting one's best foot forward versus outright deception. We're supposed to present ourselves in a positive light, obviously – nice clothes and hair, good manners, monitoring our spontaneous impulses. Wait, is this a job interview?

It might feel like we're putting up a false front, trying to trick our date into liking us. This begs the question: what's going to happen when they eventually figure out who we really are? How will they handle their inevitable disappointment? Probably by ditching us, of course.

On the other hand, maybe *they're* trying to trick us! What if they're not who or what they seem to be? Is it safe to let our guard down?

And what if we get all excited and the feelings aren't reciprocated? Ouch! Rejection is a bitch!

Sometimes it's clear to both parties right away that it's not going to work out. There's just no chemistry, and time drags by. Or maybe it's just clear to *us*. Then we're stuck having to awkwardly endure the rest of the date while coming up with a graceful enough rejection for the ending. Ugh!

Speaking of awkward, if you're going to a restaurant on a date, who pays? Is it still the guy? Or is that sexist? The rules seem much less clear these days and fraught with political correctness issues. As if things weren't complicated enough already!

What if it turns out your date just wants sex? Or perhaps *you* get overwhelmed by desire and go for it. Will you end up feeling used? And how do you feel about your date seeing you naked?

Lucky for us, online dating apps have pretty much solved all of these problems.

Ha ha, just kidding! Most apps basically require you to craft an advertising campaign for yourself and *publish* it. And perusing their profiles and messages becomes an exercise in reading between the lines. It's like having a new hobby. How fun is that?

And you'll almost certainly get "ghosted" at some point, when someone you might be into, someone you've invested time and energy in, just disappears with no explanation. Time to second-guess yourself. A whole new way to feel bad.

I've worked with quite a few women who'd developed a near *phobic* aversion to online dating. We'll get into tapping on all of this in just a bit, but first let's look at what might be the most terrifying aspect of dating: it could lead to a relationship!

Isn't a Relationship the Whole Point?

Yes, but. If your last relationship went down in flames, if you've ever been cheated on, if someone you loved became abusive or distant and cold, why on Earth would you *ever* want to put yourself through that again? Or even risk it? I mean, aside from terrible loneliness.

You wouldn't. But even if *you* decide it's worth the risk, you probably have Younger Selves who strongly disagree. Whether they're from a tragic adolescent heartbreak or some recent nightmare breakup, if losing weight is the first step toward a new relationship, they'll make damned sure *that* isn't going to happen. Looks like another possible Secret Reason.

Let's say you decide to go ahead and date *before* losing weight and meet someone you like who's totally into you. Success! Life is good! But you might still want to lose weight for any number of valid reasons. What if they prefer the heavier you and aren't interested in the skinnier version? Oh no!

Or let's say you *do* lose weight; you start dating and meet someone awesome. Perfect! You're living the dream! But what happens if you begin to put on weight again? Will they reject you? Will they become disgusted and want out? If gaining weight again seems inevitable, aren't you just signing up for inevitable heartbreak?

Making Friends with Rejection

Nobody likes being rejected, right? If we're already burdened with low self-esteem, rejection can be especially devastating. It seems to confirm our worst fears about ourselves.

Okay, so here's a crazy idea: What if you could swap out all that hurt for gratitude? Trade anguish for relief? What if you could actually make friends with romantic rejection? Ridiculous, right? Hold on, hear me out...

Let's face it, none of us are getting any younger. One of the main complaints I hear about dating is that it's a *huge* waste of time and energy. Don't you feel that way too? Well, from that perspective, rejection is a wonderful time-saver. Seriously.

If it's not going to work out with someone, wouldn't you rather find that out sooner than later? If your date is willing to do the heavy lifting, so to speak, by rejecting you, shouldn't the appropriate response be relief? They just saved you a whole lot of time and trouble. Now you get to dismiss the poor fool, turn to the Universe and shout "NEXT!"

Stand Ins

Of course, swapping out hurt for relief may be easier said than done, especially if your potential suitor is *standing in* for a parent who rejected you as a child. This is shockingly common, in my experience.

Our subconscious minds are incredibly adept at using romantic relationships to reenact childhood trauma.

Sometimes it's about the way you were treated by a parent. Sometimes it's the trauma you went through watching the train wreck of mom and dad's relationship.

Either way, reenactment is a terrible strategy for healing anything, and refusing to play along, refusing to feel hurt or rejected is great way to shut it all down.

You'll find a few lines about this in the tapping script below. If we can get you immune to the pain of rejection, this whole dating/relationship thing may become a bit more fun. Maybe.

What Can Tapping Do?

If you do have a history of painful or traumatic relationships, EFT tapping can help release the old distress and break any unwanted patterns you've been stuck with. Working with a qualified EFT practitioner is probably your best bet for really serious relationship trauma, and will likely bring about wonderful upgrades in your life.

For our more immediate purposes though, let's see if we can get your subconscious to stop using fat as protection from cupid's arrows.

Tapping for Dating and Relationship Fears

Tapping on the karate chop point:

Even if I really have been using the need to lose weight as an excuse to avoid dating or having another relationship, I totally forgive myself for that.

Tapping through the points:

I really *do* want a relationship
A good one, I mean
But there's no way I'm going to start dating until I lose weight

And yeah, I've been telling myself that for a long time
Too long maybe
But still, I really *do* need to lose weight
Seriously!
There's just no way in hell I'm putting myself out there
like this
What kind of partner would want me when I'm this fat?
Not the kind of partner I want
Yuck
There'd have to be something wrong with them
To think *this* is okay?
To think *this* is sexy?
Gross!
Not the one for me

I have to lose *at least* __ pounds before I'd put myself out
there
But to be honest, putting myself "out there" sucks
I hate it
It's such a waste of time
Even when it's obviously not going to work
I can't just say so and walk out
I have to make sure I don't hurt their stupid feelings!
Ugh, I hate it

But if we have a bunch of dates and it doesn't work out
That's even worse
It's such a stupid game
It's so phony
And most of the time they just want sex
They're just pretending to care trying to get me into bed
Ugh, all that pressure
And the skinnier I am the more *that's* going to happen
There's no way I'm going to lose weight!
I should put on *more* weight
I want to keep those users away from me!
All of this fat is protecting me

I want someone who *sees* me
Who likes me for myself
Who doesn't care about my body so much
Except *I* care
I'm not okay with my body
Maybe I want them to love me in a way I can't love myself
But then I'm going to judge the hell out of them for it?
It's like there's no way to win

And what if I'm into someone and they ghost me?
Or worse, they walk out on me?
I just can't take another rejection
It's too painful
It's devastating!
I can't put myself through that again
So thank god for all this fat
I'm never ever, ever, ever going to lose this weight
It's the only thing protecting me from myself
From putting myself out there again
Ugh!

But what if rejection didn't hurt so much?
What if it didn't hurt at all?
If I'm fooling myself into liking someone who's wrong for
me
I don't want to waste a lot of time finding out
The longer it takes to realize they suck
The more time I've wasted
And the more complicated it gets

There's no way the *right* one would reject me
If they're right, then why would they?
Even my worst qualities, they'd probably find endearing
The right one is going to be totally into me
And they're the one I want
They're the ONLY one I want
Everyone else can fuck off

So if I *do* get rejected by someone
That means they're not the right one for me!
And that's *all* it means
They just did me a big fat favor
They saved me from wasting any more time with them

They're the wrong one
I'd love to feel grateful instead of hurt
To feel nothing but relief
To forget Mr/Ms Wrong and shout "NEXT!"
And the more I love myself
The more I can just be my *real* self
The easier it will be for Mr/Ms Right to recognize me
The sooner we're likely to meet and get together

I've been hurt in the past
But I'm not the same person I was
I don't need this fat to keep me safe from getting hurt
I choose to trust myself to say no to Mr/Ms Wrong
And I choose to look forward to meeting Mr/Ms Right
They might not care how much I weigh
But I do
And I don't need this fat anymore
I don't need to be protected
I give my body permission to stop helping me
To stop helping by carrying all of this extra weight
Thank you, body, but I got this!

Younger-Self Tapping for Relationship Pain

Tapping on the karate chop point:

Even if you feel really hurt and rejected right now, that was just the wrong person at the wrong time and you are totally worthy of love and you'll find it.

Tapping through the points:

All of this pain
I know how devastating this is

I'm you from the Future
I've already gone through this and it's awful
You probably think you'll never be loved again
That maybe you're just unlovable
How could they hurt you this way?
It's so painful
All this pain
All of this heartbreak
Why didn't they love you?
How could they *do* this to you?
What's wrong with you to be treated so badly?
What did you do to deserve this?

I won't lie to you
There *is* something wrong with you
But it's not what you think
This didn't happen because you're unlovable
It happened because you picked the wrong person
I know you probably thought they were perfect
And they were
Perfect for hurting you
Perfect for breaking your heart
And that's exactly why you fell for them

I know it's twisted
But that really is why you fell for them
Your subconscious mind wants to heal you
By putting you through hell again and again
Something happened to us as kids
This person was standing in for mom/dad (or whoever)
You picked the perfect person to act just like mom/dad
This whole relationship was doomed from the start
Not because you're unlovable
You just picked the perfect person to hurt you

It isn't just you
Everyone goes through this
It's so stupid
If there's someone who really loves you

And they're *not* going to ruin your life
They probably seem boring
You probably won't look at him twice
They're standing there with a heart-shaped box of
chocolates
And a freaking bouquet of roses
But they're *boring*
They'll never turn your life into a living hell!
The exciting person is the one to do that
That's *why* they got you so excited

It's not your fault
Your subconscious did this to you
It was trying to heal you
But in the dumbest way possible
By putting you through it all over again
I'm here to help you
Let's make sure this never happens again
You were *always* worthy of love
Even if mom/dad (or whoever) did a really bad job of
loving you

You thought you loved this person
You didn't though
You loved the person you *thought* they were
They were never that person
The person you *thought* they were wouldn't have hurt you
They wouldn't have dreamed of hurting you
Basically you got tricked
Maybe they tricked you
But definitely your subconscious mind did
It was trying to heal your wounds
From mom/dad not loving you the way you needed

You don't actually need someone to do that
We can heal you right now with this tapping

You've always been worthy of love
It was *never* your fault it didn't happen

There's nothing wrong with who you are
You're a wonderful person
You're going to be loved
And the more you can love yourself
The less you actually *need* them to do it for you
The sooner the right person will show upSection Three

Breakthrough Strategies

"Whatever you are doing, love yourself for doing it. Whatever you are thinking, love yourself for thinking it. Love is the only dimension that needs to be changed. If you are not sure how it feels to be loving, love yourself for not being sure of how it feels"
--Thaddeus Golas

CHAPTER 14

Cravings

In my EFT workshops I always do a demonstration where we tap away cravings. If we're meeting in person, I bring chocolate. I always get the good stuff: organic, fair-trade and of course both milk and dark.

Before we start, I'll hand out a piece of chocolate to each person and ask them to look at it, smell it, and then rate their craving on a scale of zero to ten. Then we'll go ahead and do the tapping.

Cravings tapping often amazes people, especially if they've never done EFT before and their craving is strong. The intensity almost always drops very quickly. It can be genuinely astonishing! That said, I like to tell my students it's really more of a "parlor trick" than a serious approach to helping someone lose weight.

Unless our underlying issues (the Secret Reasons) are addressed, we'll likely just find something new to crave. I actually saw this with a client who was consuming a *quart* of Haagen-Dazs every day. We easily tapped away her craving for ice cream but then she switched to eating an extra-large pepperoni pizza instead.

Dr. Roger Callahan, the psychologist who first discovered tapping way back in the late 70s, famously said: "The true cause of addictions is anxiety—an uneasy feeling that is temporarily masked or tranquilized by some substance or behavior." For my Haagen-Dazs client, removing that anxiety meant resolving childhood sexual abuse.

Compulsions

In my own experience, craving a food doesn't always enhance enjoyment. In fact, there may be an inverse relationship. I used to have a very strong craving for chocolate. We'd buy a bar, put it up in the kitchen cabinet and sooner or later (usually sooner) I'd open the wrapper, break off a square and that first piece would be an ecstatic experience.

Of course, I'd have another and that second square might be almost as good. The third piece not so much. I'd decide "Well, that's enough for now" and go back to work, but somehow, I'd soon find myself back at the cupboard having another piece.

And then another. And another. And with each piece I'd enjoy it less and less. But the craving was compulsive! I'd eat that whole damned bar of chocolate in one day and end up not feeling very well. By the end it wouldn't even taste good. The ecstasy of that first bite devolved into actually feeling ill.

Despite all of that, I have to admit I was reluctant to tap away my craving for chocolate. Didn't matter. All of those cravings demonstrations in all of those EFT workshops did the trick, whether I wanted it to or not! Now I can take it or leave it. Instead of lasting just one day, my chocolate bars often last weeks.

Why was I so reluctant to tap away a destructive craving? Why would anyone be?

Let's face it, whatever we're indulging in tends to be pretty reliable, right? It *always* makes us feel better (at least initially). It's something we can count on. In a chaotic world, that could be a really big deal.

Whatever food we're craving probably gives us some sense of control over our own emotional state. Why on Earth would we give that up?

That's exactly the kind of resistance that can show up when we're tapping away a craving. What's so interesting though, is that we can still enjoy the food once the craving is gone. In fact, we might actually enjoy it more! Once the spell of the compulsion is lifted, we're more present, more mindful when we're eating it.

The Dog People

Getting back to my EFT workshop, we'd just keep tapping as a group until everyone's craving intensity dropped down to a zero. For some this would happen very quickly, in just a round or two. Others might take a bit longer, but it was usually a done deal in 10 to 15 minutes.

At that point I'd have everyone take a little nibble of their piece of chocolate, just to see if that spiked the craving back up, in which case we'd tap some more. Most people would say "Meh. It tastes okay, but I don't want it right now." On rare occasions though, some would actually spit it out and say "Yuck!" They might even think the chocolate bar was spoiled somehow.

I found this fascinating! In trying to get my head around this strange reaction I came to believe that for some people, maybe even most people, chocolate is harmless. It might even be good for them, at least in moderation.

But for other folks it's actually kind of toxic. I think of them as the dog people, since you're never supposed to give a dog chocolate, right? Interestingly, these were often the ones with the strongest craving.

Once that craving was tapped away, they were finally able to hear the voice of their own body. And their body was clearly saying "Yuck!" Somehow that voice had always been drowned out by the craving, which may have begun with some sort of childhood experience: "Oooh chocolate, yum yum."

Another possible source of resistance to tapping away cravings is the specter of deprivation, which we looked at in Chapter 11. I'll just mention here that there may be more going on with a craving than just the taste, texture and flavor.

Sometimes there's a deep meaning attached to that specific food or drink. An association with the rare moments your family was happy together, for example. Or times when you felt special or cared for. A memory of being comforted, perhaps associated with your "comfort food."

If your craving is stubborn and hard to tap away, exploring and tapping on possible meanings and associations with that food may help you tap your way free.

A Parlor Trick?

Over the years I've had the opportunity to help many clients tap away cravings. Some were rather run of the mill – cinnamon buns, candy, Dr. Pepper, salami, Red Bull. But some were pretty unusual. My all-time favorite was a craving for barbecue sauce! My client would take nips off the bottle, as if it were liquor. She'd polish off a whole bottle in a day or two! Happily, we were able to tap her craving away in about 15 minutes.

Although I've sometimes called it a parlor trick, tapping away a serious craving can actually be a very empowering experience. It brings feelings of mastery and hope that things can actually change.

I had a delightful German client once, born at the end of WWII. Our first three sessions tackled some serious post-war childhood trauma. At the start of our fourth session she totally surprised me, asking if I could help with her weight problem. I had no idea she *had* a weight problem (we were meeting on Skype) and told her so.

She exclaimed "Look at me!" Holding up her hands she said "Look at my fingers! They're like sausages! I'm going to explode!" She told me she felt powerless over her cravings for sweets, and there were three in particular we ended up working on.

First up was some sort of cake I'd never heard of. It came in a waxy paper box and though she'd just polished one off before our session, she still had the box with greasy crumbs stuck to the inside. That box still had a distinctive burnt sugar smell that sent craving surprisingly high. We soon had it tapped down to zero.

Next up, she had a chocolate bar on her desk. She told me she'd been having one after each of our sessions, and that was certainly her plan for this bar! Once again, her craving dropped from very high down to zero in just a few rounds. This was followed by some kind of super-expensive vegan "ice cream" in her freezer she said was calling her name. Once again, down to zero in minutes.

The following week, when the Skype picture started, she was holding up the chocolate bar with a triumphant look on her face. "Look! It's still here!" She'd had no chocolate, no cake, and the vegan ice cream hadn't been touched all week.

She had told me about her weekly trip to the grocery store where she'd push her cart down the treat isle. On one side were the cookies and cakes; on the other, ice cream and frozen desserts; and there she was, running the gauntlet, engaged in a Titanic struggle she was doomed to lose.

A few days after our previous session, she'd sauntered down that aisle, looking side to side and saying "Fuck you! Fuck you!" to all those formerly tempting treats. She laughed in delight telling me this. Victory at last!

Just a reminder, we'd already cleared quite a bit of the childhood trauma that had been troubling her. If we'd started out with the cravings, I'm not sure she'd have had such amazing results.

Limitations

A woman once asked me "Can you tap away my craving for food?" Alas, my answer was no. We can only tap away what's *not* supposed to be there, and all of us need food for sustenance. That said, we can definitely go after specific problem foods like chocolate, French bread, cookies, red wine, whatever plagues you.

As far as "too much of a good thing" though, it may be possible to tap away the craving to overeat or clean your plate. To have a second or third helping. For that particular craving, it may be easiest to tap it away when you're really feeling it. That might take a bit of planning ahead.

When tapping, it's best to go after one craving at a time. If you have lots of different cravings, choose the worst of them to start and measure the intensity of *that* craving on our zero-to-ten scale. You'll probably need to go through the tapping script more than once. Just keep going until the intensity has dropped to zero, then move on to the next craving if you like.

You might be wondering, will tapping for cravings work on more serious addictions? Like alcohol, smoking or even something like hard drugs? My answer is...maybe.

There may be Secret Reasons keeping those addictions in place that we aren't really looking at in this book. If so, they'll need to be addressed, perhaps with help from an experienced practitioner. But I don't think there's any harm in trying to tap away a craving, whatever the substance or behavior.

Tapping for Chocolate Cravings

Feel free to substitute whatever food you like.

On a scale of zero to ten, how strong is your craving right now? You might want to have the food on hand and maybe smell it to get the most accurate reading.

Tapping on the karate chop point:

Even though I have this craving for chocolate, I deeply love and completely accept myself.

Tapping around the points:

This craving
This craving for chocolate
Mmmmmm
I'd really love to eat this chocolate right now!
This craving
This craving for that rich chocolatey taste
It's so rich and smooth and sweet
I love the way it melts on the back of my tongue
This craving for chocolate
This craving

I love how I feel when I'm eating this chocolate
I love how wonderful it tastes
That rich chocolatey taste
This craving for chocolate
I'll never give this up
I'd be crazy to let this craving go
I *love* this chocolate

I know exactly how I'll feel when I eat it
Chocolate is my best friend

I can always count on chocolate
It always makes me feel better
I've always been so happy eating chocolate
There are so many happy memories
Chocolate tastes like happiness!
This craving for chocolate
This craving

I would *never* want to lose my enjoyment
But what if I could actually enjoy it more?
What if this craving doesn't add anything good?
It just makes me eat too much
I eat chocolate until it doesn't even taste good
What if I can tap away this craving
And keep loving chocolate
Or maybe love it even more?

I give myself permission to let this craving go
This craving for chocolate
This feeling that I can't get enough
This feeling that I'm under a spell
It's like I'm half asleep
I don't even enjoy it that much
I just can't stop
I can't stop craving this chocolate
And I forgive myself for that

Even if I never get over this craving for chocolate
I still deeply love and accept myself
I forgive myself
It's just so great having something I can count on
Something to control the way I feel
To make myself feel better
But I don't end up feeling better when I eat too much!
This craving
This craving to just keep eating until I'm sick
This craving for that yummy chocolate

I give myself permission to hear the voice of my own body
To hear what it wants me to eat
Or not eat
So that I can feel good all the time
Or at least most of the time
So I can enjoy the chocolate
Without needing it

CHAPTER 15

Listening to Your Body's Wisdom

Imagine you're standing in line at a deli, looking up at the menu and trying to decide what to order. On one hand, that roasted eggplant sandwich sounds great; on the other hand, maybe the Greek salad? You think "Hmmm, now what do I want?"

If you think about it, that's kind of a strange question. Who is asking, and who is being asked?

I always thought it was weird that the Royals refer to themselves as "We" instead of "I" (at least in the movies). But maybe "We" is more accurate for all of us. We definitely seem to have "parts" and sometimes different parts want different things. So, choosing what to order can be something of a negotiation.

I believe some or most of our "parts" are Younger Selves. They're all different ages and have their own preferences. The younger ones are probably clamoring for treats or comfort food. Greek salad? No way! How about a grilled cheese sandwich? Or just a great big cookie?

In the cacophony of sorting out what "We" want, one especially quiet voice can easily be missed – the voice of our physical body.

Your *body* has zero interest in emotional eating. Health and physical well-being are its imperative. Structural repair and maintenance. Vibrant energy rather than momentary pleasure.

I can testify that whenever I've heeded my body's own voice, and chosen to eat something unusual (for me), it's always tasted incredibly good. Surprisingly good! I really wasn't expecting to enjoy those steamed beets or that kale smoothie so much. I guess my body genuinely needed some particular nutrient that informed my tastebuds in a wonderful way.

Wouldn't it be great if we could amplify your body's quiet voice in any given situation? To open a direct line of communication? Allow me to share one way I've found for bypassing the clamor of the "We" and asking directly what your body wants.

Muscle Testing

Applied Kinesiology, informally known as *muscle testing*, is based on the idea that telling an *untruth* puts our body in a state of incongruence that momentarily weakens our muscles. We can take advantage of this by noticing how our muscles respond to a yes/no or true/false statement.

There are a number of ways to do muscle testing, and the one I'll be sharing here is called the Strike-Through Method. I like it because it's relatively discreet (for when you're standing in line at the deli) and offers clear results, but you can easily research other methods if this one isn't to your liking.

The Strike-Through Method:

1. With one hand make a circle with your index finger and thumb –the OK symbol.
2. Insert the index finger of your other hand into the circle.

3. Holding the OK circle lightly closed, say your True/False statement while trying to break through the circle at the point where the OK index finger and thumb meet.

If you can "strike through" the OK circle then your body recognizes the statement as FALSE. If the OK circle holds firm and you can't break through, that suggests that the statement is TRUE and in congruence with your body's wisdom.

Again, this is because a lie, false statement or untruth will temporarily weaken our muscles, or at least that's the idea.

There's a simple way of "calibrating" your finger muscles to give you accurate answers. Start by trying to strike through while saying "Yes" again and again, while making sure your finger does *not* break through the circle.

Next try saying "No" over and over, while subtly allowing your finger to slip through with each "No." This is a way of fine tuning the muscle tension in the "OK sign" hand.

Instead of saying Yes and No, you can also calibrate by making a deliberately true or false statement. For example, I might say "My name is Rob Nelson" and the OK sign stays strong – my index finger does *not* pass through. Then "My name is Mickey Mouse." This time the finger should strike through, since an untruth makes us weaker.

Once you've got your Yes/No or True/False dialed in, it's good to ask your questions as clearly as possible to avoid ambiguity. And there are certain terms like "should," "okay" and "good for me" you may want to define for yourself.

For example, the word "should" could have moral or ethical overtones: I *should* eat this fried okra just to be polite, I don't want to hurt grandma's feelings. Or I *should* eat it just to prove I'm not a vegetable-hating little kid anymore.

For our purposes, how about we define "should" as helping us lose weight or feel better in our body? Same for the word "okay" or "good for me." That way your body will be clear on the answer.

Question Authority

When it comes to asking about food and eating, I believe your body is the highest authority. With muscle testing you have a way of asking its opinion.

I've heard it said that the more you trust the answers you get, the more you act on them, the clearer the guidance becomes over time. It's a working relationship, I guess.

Just the other morning I was in my kitchen, trying to decide whether to forego coffee that day. I hate to admit it, but that was a tough decision to make. I really love my morning coffee, but coffee does not always love me back.

This was a job for muscle testing: "Can I drink coffee today without getting sick?"
A quick and easy strike through gave me the clear and emphatic answer: NO!
No coffee for me that day.

I think there's nothing wrong with comfort food in general. And there's definitely nothing wrong with the desire to *feel* comforted. But temporary comfort pales in comparison with sustained health and vitality, and for me personally, eating just the wrong thing at just the wrong time can really wipe me out. I've found muscle testing to be a great way to avoid shooting myself in the foot.

Here are examples of statements or questions I might muscle-test for:

True/False Statements

Ordering the salad is my healthiest choice.

It's okay to have second helpings.

Drinking this coffee won't keep me awake tonight.

I can eat this bread without feeling bloated.

I should go to Jenny's birthday dinner.

I need to eat before we go out.

Skipping lunch is a good idea today.

I should have steamed beets for dinner.

Yes/No Questions

Is it okay for me to eat dairy today?

Can I get away with having another cup of coffee?

Will eating this chocolate make it hard to sleep tonight?

If I eat this piece of pie, will I regret it later?

Should I have Thai food for dinner?

Do I need to drink water instead of eating?

Am I actually hungry right now?

Do I want to eat just because I'm nervous?

Test Drive

Feel free to totally disregard this whole idea of muscle testing. It's really just an adjunct to the work of clearing your Secret Reasons. But if you find it intriguing, I suggest practicing a lot. It may take a little time to open up clear lines of communication with your body.

In other words, don't wait for a crisis (like me with my morning coffee question!) to try it out.

CHAPTER 16

Tapping Away Limiting Beliefs

Have you ever had your computer glitch on you? One day I opened up my laptop, naively expecting to see the presentation I'd been working on, and was confronted instead with the dreaded Windows "blue screen of death." Oh boy, that was a rough day!

Viruses and defective software are the usual suspects with these disasters, installing faulty lines of code into the computer's operating system. The ensuing mayhem can be pretty disruptive, though usually more fixable than the "fatal error" that killed my laptop.

If you think of your brain as a kind of computer, then *beliefs* are like lines of code running in your operating system, and faulty beliefs can cause serious glitches in your life. When it comes to successfully losing weight and keeping it off, debugging your belief system can be a real game-changer.

What *Are* Beliefs?

As mentioned in Chapter 2, a belief is simply an idea that we've accepted as true and no longer question. No further evidence or verification is required. In fact, we may be inclined to disbelieve or ignore new information that contradicts our beliefs, as a way of avoiding unpleasant and unsettling "cognitive dissonance."

Being confronted with the possibility they've been wrong and having to go "back to the drawing board" can make some people really upset, sometimes even violent. Very few people seem to enjoy having their beliefs questioned or challenged.

Well, I hope *you* don't mind! This chapter is all about challenging (and hopefully changing) negative limiting beliefs about weight that may be keeping you stuck. Rather than being upset, I hope you'll be delighted by the freedom this gives you. Tossing those stale old beliefs out the window should give you a nice fresh breath of air.

Believing is Seeing

How powerful are beliefs? I'm sure you've heard of the placebo effect. Whenever new medicines are tested for efficacy, researchers have to set up two groups of patients, divided up randomly so that neither they nor the researchers know who is in which group. In fact, the test subjects may not even realize there *are* two groups.

One group, of course, receives the actual medicine being tested. The other "control group" is given a placebo – usually just an inert chalk or sugar pill.

Here's the amazing part: On average, the placebo works for about 30% of the control group. Thirty percent! Just the *belief* they are taking a real medicine actually *heals* nearly a third of the subjects. The compounds being tested have to do better than the placebo in order to be approved for use, and many fail that test.

And this isn't just for drugs. Years ago, a study was done to see which of two different knee surgeries would be more effective. In this case the patients were divided into three groups, one for each treatment and another to be the control group.

As a placebo, the control subjects were given the same local anesthetic, but the doctor simply made a small incision on their knee, no actual surgery.

Can you guess which group did the best? Not only did the control group do significantly better; *their* healing results lasted much longer. Can you see how powerful a belief can be when it comes to your own body?

Unfortunately, this effect can work both ways. With medical test results, if a patient is told they only have a few weeks to live, they might obligingly die right on schedule. This actually happens! Even when the doctor was mistakenly reading a different patient's chart.

Debugging Your Operating System

This chapter takes a direct approach to tapping away the *validity* of specific "lines of code" simply by tapping on the belief statements. Remember, the major part of your "operating system" is actually your subconscious mind, which tends to take all statements at face value. With tapping we can provide a kind of reality check, and reduce how "true" the statement feels.

If you've worked your way through the Secret Reasons chapters, many of your negative limiting beliefs about weight loss may be resolved by now. Or at least partially resolved. If so, that's great! But let's keep going and get as much of this junk out of your (operating) system as possible.

Reprogramming Your Beliefs

Here's a list of negative and limiting beliefs around weight issues. As you read through them, pay attention to how true each one feels to you. Rate each statement using a zero to one hundred percent scale.

If a statement sounds absolutely true for you then that's 100%. If it doesn't feel true at all, that's a zero. Often, it's somewhere in between. Please don't overthink your number. Honestly, whatever number comes to mind when you read the statement is the best one to use.

We're not so much interested in Universal Truth here, as much as how true the statement feels for *you* in your life right now. Because these are negative beliefs, a low number is great, and a high number means trouble.

Once you've read through the list, choose just one statement to start with. Over time you can do them all, if you like, but this process works best if you do one at a time.
And feel free to come up with statements of your own! This is not an exhaustive list. If beliefs occur to you that are not listed here, write them down and tap on them!

Limiting Beliefs Around Weight

How true are these statements for you? Please rate each one on a scale of 0 to 100%

_____ It's hard to lose weight

_____ No matter what I try, nothing ever works for me

_____ Why bother, I'll just gain it right back

_____ I'd have to give up my favorite foods; it's *so* not worth it!

_____ Now isn't a good time

_____ Some people are just naturally thin; I have fat genes

_____ I'm doomed to be fat

_____ If I were skinny, my friends would hate me

_____ If I lose weight, my mom will be sad

_____ If I lose weight, I'll get hit on, and I can't handle that

_____ To lose weight, you have to starve yourself

_____ You have to go to the gym to lose weight and I hate that!

_____ Focusing on appearance is just vanity anyway

_____ Spiritual people don't care how they look

_____ I have no self-control

_____ I can't stick with it; I can't stick with anything

_____ It's impossible to lose weight after _____ (pick an age)

_____ It's impossible to lose weight after _____ (menopause/having kids/etc.)

_____ I've never been slim, it's just not possible for me

_____ I just have a slow metabolism

Time for Some EFT

Choose one belief statement to start with and let's do some tapping! If you haven't learned EFT yet, please visit Chapter 3 for the EFT Crash Course.

The easiest way to get going is to just repeat the statement over and over, saying all or part of it for each point. After a few rounds of this, you might play with the wording, exaggerate it a bit, or focus in on some aspect of the statement that holds the most emotional charge for you. _See the example below for inspiration._

If a memory comes up while tapping, make a note of it. Perhaps it's where you first took on the belief, or maybe it's an emotionally intense incident that gave that belief special importance.

If it's a strong memory, you might take a break from tapping on the statement and instead tap on whatever feelings are coming up just from thinking about what happened. Measure the intensity of those feelings on the EFT zero to ten scale, and try tapping them down as close to zero as possible. Once the memory loses its charge, check back in on that belief statement – does it seem as true?

From Tragedy to Comedy

EFT can be *crucial* for making positive belief changes by releasing the old, stuck feelings that hold negative beliefs rigidly in place. It's wonderfully liberating to let go of beliefs that have been sabotaging you and keeping you from achieving your goals.

Often, while tapping on a negative belief, it will begin to seem absurd! Even if moments before the statement seemed completely true, suddenly it just sounds ludicrous. You might actually start laughing.

When this sudden shift happens, my guess is that we were very young when we decided that belief was true. Having little knowledge and experience of life, even the smartest kids can draw some incredibly dumb conclusions.

Remember the placebo effect? Tapping down your belief in these statements could have an actual, biological effect on your body. Get them down to 0% and watch out! You'll be giving yourself real freedom from the past.

A little tapping can go a long way, and it really doesn't take very long – maybe ten to twenty minutes for each belief. If you commit to doing one or two beliefs a day, you could work through my list in just a few weeks.

You might try setting a timer for ten minutes and just keep tapping until it dings, then measure again – how true is the statement now? Still too high? Tap for another five minutes. Lather, rinse, repeat.

Tapping Example: It's Hard to Lose Weight

Tapping on the karate chop point:

Even though it's hard to lose weight, I deeply and completely love and accept myself.

Tapping through the points:

It's so hard to lose weight!
It's always been hard for me
I have to practically starve myself
And even then it doesn't really work
It's hard to lose weight
Maybe not for everyone
But it's totally hard for me
Always has been
Always will be
There's just something about my body
I can't lose weight
It's just too hard to lose weight

And even if by some miracle I do
It comes right back on
Why is it so easy to *gain* weight?
And so hard to lose it?
It's *hard* for me to lose weight
I try and try and try and nothing works

It's just too damned hard
I can't do it

There must be something wrong with me
Something wrong with my body
I can't lose weight
It's just too hard
It's hard to lose weight

That's my story and I'm sticking to it
It's always been hard and always will be
Nothing could possibly change that
Not this stupid tapping
Not anything
It's impossible for that to change
It will never be easy for me to lose weight
It's *impossible* for it to be easy for me
The only way I could ever lose weight is through some
monumental effort
I just don't have it in me
It's too hard

It's always been hard
That's *always* been my experience
Why would I expect that to change?
It's hard to lose weight
End of story
But God I'd love to be wrong about that!
I would *love* for that to change
What if it was so easy, I didn't even have to try?
What if it just happened?
I'd get my life back
I'd have so much more energy
But that could never happen
I couldn't be wrong
What's been true in the past will always be true

Unless I've changed, I guess
What if I'm not the same person I used to be?
What if I've dropped enough emotional baggage?
What if I really am lighter inside?

And my body will somehow adapt to that
I can't believe it
It's *always* been hard to lose weight
It always will be

Unless I really am a different me
A new and better version of myself
I know that *some* people don't have to worry about weight
They can eat anything and it doesn't matter
They don't even have to try
I'm not like them, though
Or at least I've never been that way before
I would LOVE to be that way
I would love the freedom to stop thinking about it
To stop worrying about it
And have it all just happen automatically

But it's hard to lose weight
I've always known that was true
At least for me
And I would *love* to be wrong about it
It *used* to be hard
It *used* to be hard for me to lose weight
And I'm not the person I used to be
I'm tapping my way free of the past

CHAPTER 17

Affirmations

In the fall of 1984, I was 25 years old and seriously broke. My future wife and I had thrown all of our worldly possessions into my old VW van and moved up to Ashland Oregon, pretty much on a whim. Our timing was *terrible*. Housing was scarce in Ashland and jobs even more scarce. We finally found a funky old apartment over a bookstore, but scraping up the rent was a monthly challenge.

One day I was in the library, slowly making my way down an aisle looking for a book. I can't remember what I was looking for, but I'll never forget what happened next. My hands were in my pockets and there was no one else around, but somehow a book fell off the shelf and landed right at my feet. I swear I'm not making this up.

The book was Shakti Gawain's *Creative Visualization* and it was my introduction to the fascinating world of affirmations. That book triggered a much-needed upgrade to our prosperity as a couple.

What Are Affirmations?

In the last chapter we looked at negative limiting beliefs. Affirmations are pretty much just the opposite: positive statements intended to *expand* our outlook on the good things that are possible. Affirmations are ideas that you probably don't believe but would very much like to.

Why? If you can somehow get an affirmation accepted as unquestionable truth by your powerful subconscious mind, it's bound to improve your life. You'll begin to perceive new opportunities and possibilities. What may have seemed impossible becomes easy and automatic. Which is lovely when it comes to losing weight.

When I was broke living in Ashland, the money affirmations I tried really seemed to work. My financial situation improved almost immediately. Looking back, I don't think I had any real resistance to these new ideas about prosperity. I'd just never encountered them before. Unfortunately, it's not always so easy.

The Problem with Affirmations

Affirmations are wonderful, but how do we get our subconscious to accept them? The standard procedure is to simply repeat them over and over, ideally out loud, boldly and enthusiastically declaring them. Does this actually work? Not very often and not very well, at least for most of us.

Whenever we have countervailing beliefs, especially if they're emotionally charged and based on some kind of negative lived experience, affirmations don't really stand a chance. However much we'd like to believe them, our subconscious mind is having none of it. Its prime directive is to keep us safe, mainly by projecting our past onto the future. Not a lot of wiggle room there for positive change.

For example, you might *love* the affirmation "It is safe, fun and appropriate to become more and more attractive." On a rational level that might be very appealing, and very helpful for losing weight.

Unfortunately, there may have been a time in your past when it was anything but safe or fun to be attractive. Some ugly experience may have made you intensely uncomfortable and led your Younger Self to make the decision that being attractive was actually dangerous. Can you see how no amount of enthusiastic repetition is going to override that experience?

That's exactly the point of going through the Secret Reasons, or at least the ones relevant to you. Addressing and resolving those directly can effectively prepare the subconscious to allow changes. It's kind of like having a garden bed full of noxious weeds. They definitely need to be pulled out before planting the beautiful flowers we'd like to see. Or, in this case, *implanting* lovely new affirmations we'd like to believe.

That said, if you've skipped straight to this chapter, I suggest you stop and go back to the Secret Reasons section first. Doing so will almost certainly make this chapter *much* more effective.

Tapping is the Game Changer

EFT tapping communicates directly with your non-verbal, emotional brain, releasing old stuck negative feelings and beliefs. In tapping for affirmations, our focus is on removing any resistance or obstacles your subconscious may have to accepting them.

Having already done significant work on our Secret Reasons, much of that subconscious resistance may be gone, and we'll just be mopping up whatever is left. The method that is easiest to put into practice is to tap through the points while simply saying the affirmation over and over. The assumption with that approach is that objections will be automatically released even if we're not aware of what they are.

This is definitely the most simple and direct approach, though maybe not the most effective. Another option is to frame the affirmation negatively and target potential blocks directly.

For example: "Even though I'd *love* to believe that I can easily reach and maintain my ideal weight, I know it's just not true for me. But I still deeply love and completely accept myself."

With this more negative approach, it's a good idea to tap on every single reason the affirmation feels untrue. This might seem counterproductive, but you can't trick the subconscious by pretending these things aren't real. Even when the objections are valid, tapping can still work magic by removing some of the negative emotional charge.

See the example below for inspiration.

How to Proceed

As you read through this list of affirmations, pay attention to how true each one feels for you. Rate each statement using a zero to one hundred percent scale.

If a statement sounds totally true for you then that's one hundred percent. If it doesn't feel true at all, that's a zero. Often, it'll be somewhere in between. Don't overthink it; as with tapping for negative beliefs, whatever number comes to mind when you read the statement is the best one to use.

We're not so much interested in Universal Truth here, it's more a question of how true the statement is for *you* in your life right now. Because these are positive statements, the higher your number the better. If you're already at 100% there's really no need to tap on that particular affirmation.

Once you've gone through the list, choose just one affirmation to start with. You might start with one that has the lowest number, or perhaps one really stands out for you. Over time you can do them all, and ideally get every one of them up to 100%, but this process works best if you do one at a time. This is not an exhaustive list by any means, so feel free to add any affirmations you'd like.

Weight Affirmations

How true are these statements for you?

_____ My weight-loss journey is a joyful experience.

_____ My metabolism is now set for my ideal weight of ____ pounds.

_____ Unhealthy foods no longer appeal. My body craves health and vitality!

_____ I can easily reach and maintain my ideal weight.

_____ My body knows what it needs, and that's all I'm hungry for.

_____ I feel safe and comfortable having a lean, healthy, and attractive body.

_____ I enjoy attention and admiration from others.

_____ It is safe, fun and appropriate to become more and more attractive.

_____ I'm proud of setting a good example for my family and friends.

_____ I love and accept my body as it is, and as it changes.

_____ I've let go of any guilt I have around food.

_____ I show my body gratitude by nourishing it with healthy foods.

_____ Every part of me wants to be slim, healthy and beautiful.

_____ I love all parts of my body.

_____ I look in the mirror and like what I see.

_____ I'm always kind to my body.

_____ I allow myself to feel good being me.

_____ I gracefully release relationships that no longer support my highest and best life.

_____ I am loved and supported on my weight-loss journey

_____ I nurture my physical body in healthy and loving ways.

Let's Get Tapping

Once you've decided on one affirmation to start with and you've measured how true it seems, let's do some tapping. If you haven't learned EFT yet, please visit Chapter 3 for the EFT Crash Course.

As you tap, if any memories, limiting beliefs, or blocks come up, please make note of them, maybe even stopping to write them down. If it's emotionally charged, you might want to take a break from the affirmation tapping to address whatever it is directly, tapping away whatever negative charge it might have.

For any given affirmation, it might only take ten to twenty minutes of tapping to really start believing it's true. For some it might take longer, but doing just one a day, you'll power through this list in less than a month.

Will this really help you lose weight and keep it off? Let's find out!

Tapping Script for "I can easily reach and maintain my ideal weight"

As mentioned above, you can simply repeat the statement over and over while tapping, but since you don't need a script to do that, here's an example putting the affirmation in a negative context, in order to harness the awesome power of EFT as effectively as possible.

Tapping on the karate chop point:

Even though it's just not true that 'I can easily reach and maintain my ideal weight', I really *wish* it was true for me and I forgive myself for having all of this struggle.

Tapping through the points:

It's just not true that 'I can easily reach and maintain my ideal weight'
It's never been true and never will be
Losing weight is incredibly hard for me
And even if I somehow manage it, I know it will come right back on
I *wish* it was easy but it's not
It's *not* easy to reach and maintain my ideal weight
It may not be impossible, but it's definitely not easy
No one knows how hard it's been for me
How hard I've had to struggle
And what do I have to show for it?

It's always been really hard to lose any weight
And I need to lose *so much* to reach my ideal weight
I can't even imagine how that's going to happen
The way it's been in the past is the only way it can ever be
And that's *never* been easy
Just saying "I can easily reach and maintain my ideal weight" is a joke

It's a total lie
It would have happened by now
It would have happened a long time ago
I've worked and struggled for so long and it's *never* been easy

But wouldn't it be great if it was?
Wouldn't it be so wonderful to reach my ideal weight with no struggle?
To maintain it there with no problem?
I wish it was true, that 'I can easily reach and maintain my ideal weight'
But it just isn't
Or at least it's never been true before
Something would *really* have to change for it to be easy
It would have to be a *huge* change
Almost like I'd have to be a different person
But maybe I *have* changed
Maybe I *am* a different person now
I know I'm not the same person I was ten years ago
Or even two years ago
I've changed so much even in these last few weeks

There are *reasons* it hasn't been easy to lose weight
Or at least there were reasons
It's not because I'm weak
There's been a terrible conflict over being skinnier
What if that conflict is over?
What if there's no more reason to stay fat?
I'd love to believe that 'I can easily reach and maintain my ideal weight'
I'd love for that to be true
What if all this work I'm doing is *making* it come true?
What if it's already become easier?
Part of me thinks it's crazy to believe it could ever be easy
And I forgive that part of me

I forgive my body and subconscious mind for trying to keep me safe

I *am* safe now and I allow myself to feel that
It's becoming easier and easier to feel safe
Of course 'I can easily reach and maintain my ideal
weight'
That's absolutely true for me now
I can easily reach and maintain my ideal weight

CHAPTER 18

Conclusion

"In life, understanding is the booby prize."
--Werner Erhard

The fact that you're reading this book suggests (to me at least) that you must have a superior intellect! I do hope you've picked up some useful ideas and life-changing perspectives going through these pages. However, I'm afraid Mr. Erhard is correct, as far as the booby prize goes.

If you've made it all the way to this last chapter without doing any of the tapping, you'll need to *go back and actually tap* through the relevant scripts to get the change you want.

Why? No matter how brilliant your conscious, rational mind may be, when it comes to your weight it's your *subconscious* mind running the show, and EFT tapping is an incredibly effective way of getting through to it. Words alone are pretty much useless in this regard.

So is self-discipline, alas. If you've struggled with your weight for very long, odds are you've judged yourself at times as weak-willed and undisciplined. It's easy enough to jump to that conclusion when you know what NOT to eat but go ahead and eat it anyway.

Even so, in my experience those judgements are unfair and totally unhelpful. The settings for your appetite and metabolism are actually subconscious, buried deep beneath the reach of conscious rational intentions. Trying to override those settings with will-power alone is like trying to swim against the tide.

You're not weak-willed, but rather, overmatched.

Changing the Settings

In this book we've explored seven of the Secret Reasons your subconscious may have for keeping you heavy:

- The compulsion to reenact intolerable feelings, such as shame or failure
- Protection from unwanted sexual attention
- Fear of losing important relationships, or even your identity
- Rebellion against a domineering parent/determination to win a power struggle
- A deep-down fear of deprivation, stemming from a childhood experience
- Distraction from stepping into your life in a powerful, authentic way
- An excuse to avoid dating and/or new relationships

While it's unlikely you have more than one or two of these Secret Reasons running in your subconscious, it really just takes one to override your most ardent desire to slim down. All of these reasons, each in their own way, are a *really* big deal for the subconscious, whose top priority is keeping you safe.

If keeping you safe means keeping you heavy, to your subconscious mind, that will seem like a small price to pay. The Secret Reasons may be based on traumas or bad experiences from your past, but for the subconscious mind everything is present tense. Thanks to the Freeze

Response, it's all still happening right now, just below the surface of your awareness.

EFT tapping is *the* essential change agent here. Tapping bypasses the conscious rational mind, directly accessing your subconscious emotional brain. The words we use while tapping help to dredge up the old distress so it can finally be released in the here and now.

A Great Starting Point

Resolving your old emotional junk will begin turning the tide, shutting down the relentless "undertow" you've been swimming against. And the best starting place for this is addressing whatever self-loathing or self-hate you may be harboring.

Any amount of self-hate is absolutely counterproductive. Overeating is often an attempt to find comfort and distraction, not just from the harshness of life, but from our own self-cruelty.

Self-loathing may also cause a kind of separation or dissociation from your own body, when feelings of self-disgust, shame or contempt are overwhelming. Unfortunately, the less you're able to inhabit your body, the less influence you'll have with it, and the more out of control and compulsive your eating is likely to be.

In EFT we generally balance whatever issue we're focusing on with the affirmation "I deeply love and completely accept myself," and this statement gets right to the heart of a seeming paradox: if I love myself the way I am, won't I lose my motivation to change? As strange as it may seem, the answer is no!

It's definitely possible to "hate yourself thin" but you probably know from experience that that effort is ultimately doomed. You *will* gain it all back and then some. That's why EFT is a game-changer. With tapping you can actually lose the hate for real. Lose the hate and you can win the struggle for good.

Swapping Out Old Beliefs

Your beliefs play a major role in your experience of reality, including the physical manifestation of your body.

Releasing negative emotions is incredibly helpful, and aside from helping you lose weight, it will make your life better overall. But in this book, we've gone even further by working on replacing the negative limiting beliefs you may have running in your subconscious "operating system."

The beliefs causing you the most trouble stem from decisions made by your Younger Selves, in the context of terrible experiences.

No matter how off-base or self-destructive those decisions may be in your life today, and despite being made by a young child with limited information and experience, they may seem perfectly reasonable to your subconscious mind.

Tapping is a fantastic way of getting your subconscious to change its mind about these beliefs, and that's a major goal in all of the tapping scripts in this book. Chapters 16 & 17 tackle potential belief issues head on.

Just imagine how much easier it will be for you to lose weight and keep it off once you go from believing "It's hard to lose weight" to totally *knowing* that "My weight loss journey is a joyful experience."

Your Body is the Expert

As promised, there's nothing in this book about diet or exercise (and I hope that's a relief). Your own body is the ultimate authority on what and how much you should be eating and moving at any given time. By clearing away the background noise of the Secret Reasons, my hope is that you'll hear the voice of your body with ever-increasing clarity.

To help you along with that, in Chapter 15 we took a look at using muscle testing as a means of direct communication with your body's intelligence. I hope you'll find this fascinating and kind of fun!

Major Trauma

The tapping scripts in this book have the somewhat limited objective of getting your weight out of the equation when it comes to dealing with the past. In other words, getting your subconscious to let go of weight as protection or as the solution to issues that no longer apply.

If your Secret Reasons involve really serious trauma, this book is *not* a substitute for working with a skilled EFT practitioner. You'll find a link to EFT practitioner resources in the back of this book.

That said, my hope is that going through the relevant scripts, perhaps over and over, will seriously "take the edge off" enough for your subconscious to change its mind about keeping you heavy. Once that happens, dropping down to your ideal weight tends to become automatic and inevitable.

The outcome I'm wishing for you is a wonderful lightness of being, not only for your physical weight, but in every area of your life. I love the phrase "weight loss journey" because it really can take you into new territory – happier, more successful, creative and authentically you.

Tapping Script from Hell

Note: If you've skipped to this section without learning EFT yet, I highly recommend going through the Chapter 3 "EFT Crash Course" first.

This script was given to me years ago by a dear friend who lost 40 pounds simply by tapping on these words at least once a day. There's a lot of extreme self-loathing and raw emotional intensity in this script. She didn't hold back!

I'm offering it here as an optional, additional resource. If it's too intense for you, feel free to skip the whole thing!

Like any script, some of these lines may not apply to you. It won't hurt anything to read through them anyway, or simply skip them if you like. Other lines may have a strong charge for you. You might repeat those lines over and over through multiple tapping points.

If you tap on this script daily for a while, your emotional charge is likely to diminish over time, eventually getting to zero. That's what we're after!

What Have You Got to Lose?

Tapping on the karate chop point:

Even though I have this hideous ugly fat all over my body and I feel completely trapped with it, like I'll always be an ugly fat person and a weak-willed failure, I deeply love and completely accept myself anyway.

Tapping through the points:

I really need to lose this weight *right now*!
I feel so fat and lumpy and ugly
My clothes feel so tight and my stomach is so blobby
I've been struggling with my weight forever
Seems like my whole life
And I'm afraid I'll *never* be in control

I am so attached to controlling my eating
I have this need to change the way I eat
If I don't get control, I'll just stay fat forever
Or worse, get even heavier

Only people who are lean and fit can really be happy.
I can't be happy until I weigh _____ pounds
But I am really struggling with my eating habits
I keep saying that I need to lose weight
But then I keep right on eating starch and fat and sweets,
ugh! Why??

I have this excess weight and it's just not fair!
I wish so much that I didn't have this ugly fat
Other people don't have this problem!
I really MUST lose this weight
I never feel thin enough
I *need* to lose weight now
I can't be happy with my body until I weigh under _____
pounds
I can't be happy until I have a firm, lean, healthy body

How can I feel OK with all this extra fat hanging around?
Every time I look at myself in the mirror naked, I feel
utter despair
So ugly!! Who could possibly find me attractive??

When I feel this ugly, of course I need to lose weight!
I will *not* allow myself to be happy until I have lost this
extra weight
People are crazy to tell me I'm attractive now

To be happy now, even though I have this obvious fat
problem?
My thighs are heavy
My belly rolls sticking over my waistband
My upper arms all blobby, yuck!
Only thin people can be happy

I have become really attached to wanting to be thin
I feel that I'm getting older and will never be lean in my
whole life!!
What defeat!
Being lumpy and blobby makes getting older feel so much
worse
I feel so out of control!

This tapping is NOT going to help me lose weight
How can it?
It's ineffective at best
Weird hippy clap trap. I feel so stupid doing this
What I really need to do is get an iron grip on my life
I'll have to seriously cut back on my eating
And get into some strenuous exercise to lose this weight

But I just can't get motivated
I'm naturally sedentary so I'm screwed
I don't want to have to change anything I do to lose weight
No one can tell me what to do!!
I pride myself on being a rebel
I shouldn't have to do what ordinary people do to lose
weight
I'm SPECIAL!!
Why do I have this deep block to attaining a trim
figure???
Which I must have because...I'm fat!!

There's no way I'm giving up the pleasure of beautiful
sensual food
But WHY do I eat more than my body needs?
I'll never be able to change my eating habits

And actually, deep down, I guess I don't really want to
But what if I only ate exactly what my body wanted, when
it needed it?
What would that be like?
But it's impossible to just lose weight just like that!
I'll have to starve myself to be able to lose any weight
And when I can't stand depriving myself anymore
I'll just eat my way back to being fat, as usual
Typical scenario
It's happened again and again
That's just the way it goes with me

Why do I have this deep resistance to losing these last
pounds?
If it's so easy to lose weight then why can't I just do it like
other people?
Do I breathe more air than I need?
Do I drink more water than I need?
What if I only ate exactly what my body wanted, when it
needed it?
What would that feel like?
I think I'm ready to try it out
Yes, I am ready

Why do I carry this extra weight?
What if I have a deeply submerged program inside me
that keeps me fat for some reason?
Maybe even a good reason?
Could this unsightly fat be a protection?
Maybe I unconsciously keep it on as sort of a safe suit?
Maybe when I was younger, I decided that having this
extra weight was a very good idea
Maybe even a life-saving positive thing

But I'm all grown up now. I am mature
I am now perfectly capable of protecting myself without
this extra fat hanging around
I'm strong now and can defend myself without this stupid
fat suit

This thick middle, these big thighs, these ugly lumps
I don't need them any longer

I choose to release my blocks to losing weight right now
I can be happy with myself the way I am right now
Extra weight and all
Instead of feeling fat I choose to feel healthy
I now choose to release this excess weight easily and
effortlessly
I don't even have to consciously think about it
I am reprogramming my subconscious right now for lean
healthy beauty
No more overweight issues
I let all my weight issues go now
I deserve to be happy and healthy and lean!

I am completely detached from ever needing to diet again
I don't need to control my eating anymore
I let that go
It would be nice to weigh my ideal weight right now but I
do not *need* to
I am happy right now
I am already becoming leaner every day, in every way
I do *not* need to be perfectly trim and lean to feel happy
with my body right now
I now choose to be happy and healthy instead of
discouraged about my body
Wow! I feel so free right now

I picture this fat melting away
I see it melting like ice in the hot sun because I no longer
need it
Easily
Effortlessly
I want to thank it
Yes, *thank it* for keeping me safe all these long hard years
But I no longer require its services
I really and truly don't!
I let it go now

I am letting it go
Shedding this extra weight like chaff from a seed
I no longer need it for protection

It is safe to lose weight and be visible
It is safe to lose weight and attract attention.

I was just a child when I chose to be fat
I understand now and I forgive myself
I can let go
I have real choices
I am no longer trapped

I choose to release this heaviness and this padding
I don't need it anymore
I can be perfectly safe without it
I am safe
I am open to fully blossoming in my life
I don't need to "weight" any longer

I eat only what my body needs to stay perfectly healthy and fit
I can now revel in my slim smooth belly, my firm thighs, trim hips and graceful arms
I can look at myself naked and I feel good
I like what I see
I love my beautiful body
I am so grateful for its gracious physical being
I am powerful and safe and seen in the world
My "weight" is over
I am visible and healthy and lean and beautiful!!!

Resources

Books:

Hacking Reality
by Rob Nelson

How Not to Cry
by Steph Dodds

Tap, Taste, Heal
by Marcella Friel

The Biology of Belief
by Bruce Lipton

8 Keys to Brain Body Balance
by Robert Scaer

You Can Heal Your Life
by Louise Hay

You Tube:

Tapping the Matrix (my channel)

Tapping with Steph

Surviving Narcissism

Miss Manifesther

Finding a Qualified EFT Practitioner:
tappingthematrixacademy.com/eft-practitioner-directory

Low-Cost EFT Clinic:
tappingthematrixacademy.com/academy-clinic

Acknowledgments

I have endless gratitude for Gary Craig, the founder of EFT, who generously gifted EFT to the world, and in the process, launched me into the career of my dreams. Without Gary's amazing teaching, the incredible healing represented in this book would never have happened.

Special thanks to my editors: Krista Brown and Tom Wallace. The book is *vastly* better, thanks to your diligent and brilliantly perceptive efforts.

To my wonderful clients, who trusted me with their weight loss journey (or adventure!) I'm deeply grateful. Time after time, their ardent desire to lose weight led us into deep realms of personal transformation.

To Steph Dodds, my EFT colleague and swap-partner extraordinaire, I'm very grateful. You played an important role in the realization of this book, through inspiration and by helping me shed so many obstacles to writing and publishing again.

To Joe Vitale, who liked my book Hacking Reality and told me I *had* to write more books, thank you! I believed you, and so here we are.

To Karl Dawson, creator of Matrix Reimprinting, for being such a brilliant teacher.

And special thanks to Wendy Frado, Meg Amor and Kathy Vogel for such generous, keen-eyed, volunteer proofreading!

And last but not least, I'd like to acknowledge *you*, dear reader, for your determination to have a better life, and for giving this weird tapping thing a shot. Though we'll likely never meet, you are the reason I wrote this book. Thank you for reading it!

About the Author

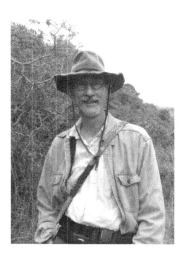

Rob Nelson, author of *Hacking Reality*, holds a Masters in Counseling Psychology and is an ordained minister in the Universal Life Church. He spent most of his early career working with traumatized children and teens, and teaching parent education classes. For a time Rob also worked the "graveyard shift" for a suicide prevention hotline.

Rob encountered EFT in 2007 and began a private practice, working with clients worldwide. He was trained and certified in EFT by Gary Craig, the founder of this modality.

As the director of Tapping the Matrix Academy, Rob also trains, mentors and certifies practitioners in EFT and his own Hacking Reality Technique.

Married since 1985, Rob has two grown daughters and makes his home in Santa Rosa, California.

www.TappingtheMatrix.com
www.instagram.com/tappingthematrix

PRAISE FOR HACKING REALITY

Engaging, intriguing, funny, and wonderfully readable...I couldn't put this book down! Stories of ordinary people creating incredible change, how they did it, and how anyone can. Rob Nelson has a real knack for explaining the science behind it all, so you'll understand and even laugh out loud. A welcome addition to the quantum consciousness field. -- Ivonne Plankey

This is definitely one of the best self-help books I've ever read. As a psychologist, I wish academics would explain things in such a simple and pleasant to read way as Rob does. The book is filled with great analogies and case examples that are used to break down complex concepts from fields such as epigenetics, quantum physics, morphogenetic fields, energy psychology, Emotional Freedom Techniques and Matrix Reimprinting. I really enjoyed reading this book and learned a lot from it. --Bruno Sade

Super interesting and fun to read, this book can turn your reality right side up. In a witty, casual style, the author explains the physics and methods of how we can rewrite experiences and beliefs that hold us back from being all of who we would like to be. I'm a counsellor with over 20 years' experience specializing in working with trauma, anxiety, depression as well as other life challenges, and I'd recommend this book to anyone! --Lieneke Hewlett

While we have all read multiple self-help books over the years, HACKING REALITY actually delivers! Rob Nelson has provided the reader with actual (and easy to learn) tools to delve deep into the subconscious and clear out old programming. Have you always felt that something holds you back or sabotages your success in life, love and dreams? Hacking Reality shows you how to live the life you always wished you had. I relished every page...his insights in what drives us through life and his gift of helping us find a new and happier path is life changing. This is a beautiful book and Rob's genuine love of helping people heal comes through on every page. --lilrose

Hacking Reality

Enjoyed Seven Secret Reasons? Check *this* out!

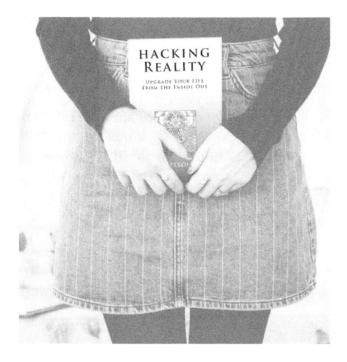

PS

I hope you've enjoyed Seven Secret Reasons and will find it genuinely helpful on your weight loss journey. If so, please consider writing a short review on whatever site you purchased the book.

Reviews are absolutely crucial for any book's success these days. I would love for readers who might benefit from Seven Secret Reasons to be able to find it! Even a line or two might make all the difference.

Thank you so much!

.

Made in the USA
Las Vegas, NV
16 November 2023

80927395R00121